URINALYSIS AND BODY FLUIDS

A SELF-INSTRUCTIONAL TEXT

87B EAST HILLSI
SOMER, NY
10589
914 277 4053

URINALYSIS AND BODY FLUIDS

A SELF-INSTRUCTIONAL TEXT

SUSAN KING STRASINGER, D.A., M.T. (A.S.C.P.)

DIRECTOR
MEDICAL LABORATORY TECHNICIAN PROGRAM
NORTHERN VIRGINIA COMMUNITY COLLEGE
ALEXANDRIA, VIRGINIA

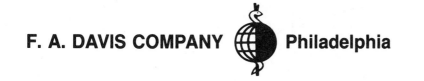

F. A. DAVIS COMPANY Philadelphia

Copyright © 1985 by F. A. Davis Company

Second printing 1985

Printed in the United States of America

Library of Congress Cataloging in Publication Data
Strasinger, Susan King.
  Urinalysis and body fluids.

  Includes bibliographies and index.
   1. Urine—Analysis. 2. Body fluids—Analysis.
3. Diagnosis, Laboratory. I. Title. [DNLM: 1. Body
Fluids—analysis—programmed texts. 2. Urine—analysis—
programmed texts. QY 18 S897u]
RB53.S87 1985   616.07′566   84-23824
ISBN 0-8036-8101-1

TO HARRY, MY EDITOR-IN-CHIEF

PREFACE

Although examination of urine was the beginning of laboratory medicine, the focus of modern clinical laboratories centers on the analysis of blood and the identification of microorganisms. Much less emphasis is placed on the testing of urine and other body fluids, even though they often provide the earliest or most specific diagnostic information. This same pattern also extends to medical technology training and the availability of student-oriented educational materials. The objective of this text is to provide students and laboratory personnel with consolidated yet comprehensive information on the analysis and clinical significance of urine, body fluids, gastric contents, and feces. Because these topics must often be covered within a limited time-frame, this text is designed for both traditional and self-instructional teaching methods. Each chapter is preceded by instructional objectives. Discussions are reinforced by diagrams, charts, and summaries. Review questions and case histories conclude each chapter.

Because many medical technology students begin their training with the study of urinalysis, the first six chapters are devoted to this subject. Chapter 1 is an introduction to urine testing. Chapter 2 covers renal physiology, renal function testing, and renal diseases. The next three chapters provide an in-depth discussion of the physical, chemical, and microscopic examinations that are performed during the routine urinalysis. The relationships among the results obtained in these three areas are stressed. Special testing procedures that are performed in the urinalysis laboratory are covered in Chapter 6. These include screening tests for aminoaciduria, porphyrias, and meliturias.

The remaining four chapters cover cerebrospinal fluid, semen, synovial fluid, serous fluids, amniotic fluid, sweat, gastric contents, and feces. Physiology, specimen collection and handling, routine and specific laboratory tests, and disease correlations are discussed for each specimen. To accommodate curriculum variations in the sequence in which various topics are introduced, the presentations on cerebrospinal fluid, synovial fluid, and serous fluids are clearly separated into sections covering the tests performed in the hematology, chemistry, microbiology, and serology laboratories. Analysis of semen, differentiation between transudates and exudates, and amniotic fluid tests for fetal well-being and maturity are discussed in detail. Methodology and calculations associated with the measurement of gastric acidity are thoroughly covered in Chapter 9. The book concludes with a chapter on fecal analysis that emphasizes tests for "occult blood" and fecal fat.

Susan King Strasinger

ACKNOWLEDGMENTS

I wish to express my appreciation to Drs. E. Kennedy, J. Rees, and C. Matta for their guidance and careful review of the manuscript, and to Dr. Renata Greenspan for her suggestions on pertinent material that should be included. The artistic contributions of Ms. Iris Denney provide a valuable addition to the text, as does the hemoglobin degradation diagram from Dr. Delia Barreto. Urinary sediments for the color plates were provided by Mr. Sherwood Bramley and Mr. Sam Yoon. Photography was performed with the assistance of Ms. Julie Johnson. Additional color plates were contributed by Mrs. Kathryn Wright and Ms. Michele Best.

Susan King Strasinger

CONTENTS

LIST OF COLOR PLATES

1
INTRODUCTION TO URINALYSIS

INSTRUCTIONAL OBJECTIVES

Upon completion of this chapter, readers will be able to:

1. list three major chemical constituents of urine
2. describe a method for determining that a questionable fluid is urine
3. list three basic rules for specimen handling and explain their importance
4. briefly discuss five methods for preserving urine specimens, including their advantages and disadvantages
5. list eight changes that may take place in a urine specimen that remains at room temperature for more than 2 hours
6. instruct a patient in the correct procedure for collecting a timed urine specimen
7. describe the type of specimen needed to obtain optimal results when a specific urinalysis procedure is requested
8. define the common terms encountered in urinalysis and use them in proper context
9. recognize common abbreviations associated with urinalysis and tell what they represent

HISTORY AND IMPORTANCE

The analysis of urine was actually the beginning of laboratory medicine. References to the study of urine can be found in the drawings of the cavemen and in Egyptian hieroglyphics such as the Edwin Smith Surgical Papyrus. Pictures of early physicians, called "pisse prophets," commonly showed them examining a glass or flask of urine. Often, these physicians never saw the patient, only the patient's urine. Although these physicians lacked the sophisticated testing mechanisms now available, they were able to obtain diagnostic information from such basic observations as color, turbidity, odor, volume, viscosity, and even sweetness, since certain specimens attracted ants. It is interesting to note that these same urine characteristics are still reported by laboratory personnel today. However, modern urinalysis has expanded its scope to include not only the physical examination of urine, but also chemical analysis and microscopic examination of the urinary sediment.

Many well-known names in the history of medicine are associated with the study of urine, including Hippocrates, who, in the fifth century BC, wrote a book on "uroscopy." Physicians concentrated their efforts very heavily on the art of "uroscopy." By 1140 AD, color charts had been developed that described the significance of 20 different colors. Chemical testing progressed from "ant-testing" and "taste-testing" for glucose to Frederik Dekkers' discovery, in 1694, of albuminuria by boiling urine and on to the measurement of such substances as gold, silver, and lead in urine in the 1800s.[5] The invention of the microscope in the 17th century led to the examination of urinary sediment and to the development by Thomas Addis of methods for quantitating the microscopic sediment. Urinalysis was introduced as part of a doctor's routine patient examination by Richard Bright in 1827. However, by the 1930s, the number and complexity of the tests performed in a urinalysis had reached a point of impracticality, and the urinalysis began to disappear from routine examinations. Fortunately, the development of modern testing techniques rescued the routine urinalysis, and it has remained an integral part of the patient examination.

Two unique characteristics of a urine specimen can account for this continued popularity:

1. Urine is a readily available and easily collected specimen.
2. Urine contains information about many of the body's major metabolic functions, and this information can be obtained by simple laboratory tests.

These characteristics fit in well with the current trends toward preventive medicine and lower medical costs. By offering an inexpensive way to test large numbers of people not only for renal disease, but also for the asymptomatic beginnings of conditions such as diabetes mellitus and liver disease, the urinalysis is a very valuable metabolic screening procedure. However, care must be taken in the laboratory not to let the simplicity of the procedure and the frequency of requests result in a relaxation of testing standards.

FORMATION

Urine is continuously formed by the kidneys. It is actually an ultrafiltrate of plasma from which glucose, amino acids, water, and other substances essential to body metabolism have been reabsorbed. The physiologic process by which approximately 170,000 ml of filtered plasma is converted to the average daily urine output of 1200 ml is discussed in detail in Chapter 2.

COMPOSITION

In general, urine consists of urea and other organic and inorganic chemicals dissolved in water. However, considerable variations in the concentrations of these substances can occur owing to the influence of factors such as dietary intake, physical activity, body metabolism, endocrine function, and even body position. Urea, a metabolic waste product produced in the liver from the breakdown of protein and amino acids, accounts for nearly half of the total dissolved solids in urine. Other organic substances include primarily creatinine and uric acid. The major inorganic solid dissolved in urine is chloride, followed by sodium and potassium. Small or trace amounts of many additional inorganic chemicals are also present in urine. The concentrations of these inorganic compounds are greatly influenced by dietary intake, making it difficult to establish normal levels. Table 1-1 shows the major chemical substances in urine. Other substances found in urine include hormones, vitamins, and medications. Although not a part of the original plasma filtrate, the urine may also contain formed elements such as cells, crystals, mucus, and bacteria. Increased amounts of these formed elements are often indicative of disease. Should it be necessary to determine if a particular fluid is actually urine, the specimen can be tested for its urea and creatinine content. Since both of these substances are present in much higher concentrations in urine than in other body fluids, the demonstration of a high urea and creatinine content can identify a fluid as urine.[2]

TABLE 1-1. Composition of Urine*

Component	Amount		Urine/Plasma Ratio
Acid	pH Ave 6.0 (range ~4.7–8.0)		
Osmolarity (mosmoles/liter)		750–1400	
Specific gravity		1.015–1.038	
Sodium	2–4 g	100–200 mEq	0.8–1.5
Potassium	1.5–2.0 g	50–70 mEq	10–15
Magnesium	0.1–0.2 g	8–16 mEq	
Calcium	0.1–0.3 g	2.5–7.5 mEq	
Iron	0.2 mg		
Ammonia	0.4–1.0 g N	30–75 mEq	
H^+		$4 \times 10^{-8} - 4 \times 10^{-6}$ mEq/liter	1–100
Uric acid	0.80–0.2 g N		20
Amino acids	0.08–0.15 g N		
Hippuric acid	0.04–0.08 g N		
Chloride		100–250 mEq	0.8–2
Bicarbonate		0–50 mEq	0–2
Phosphate	0.7–1.6 g P	20–50 mmol	25
Inorganic sulfate	0.6–1.8 g S	40–120 mEq	50
Organic sulfate	0.06–0.2 g S		
Urea	6–18 g N		35
Creatinine	0.3–0.8 g N		70
Peptides	0.3–0.7 g N		

*The values indicate the average contents of adult human urine collected for 24 h. From White, A., et al: *Principles of Biochemistry,* ed 6. McGraw-Hill, New York, 1977, p. 514, with permission.

VOLUME

Urine volume is dependent upon the amount of water excreted by the kidneys. Water is a major body constituent; therefore, the amount excreted is usually determined by the body's state of hydration. Factors that influence urine volume include: fluid intake; fluid loss from nonrenal sources; variations in the secretion of antidiuretic hormone; and the necessity to excrete increased amounts of dissolved solids, such as glucose or salts. Taking these factors into consideration, it can be seen that although the average daily urine output is 1200 to 1500 ml, a range of 600 to 2000 ml may be considered normal.[2]

Oliguria, a decrease in the normal daily urine volume, is commonly seen when the body enters a state of dehydration due to excessive water loss from vomiting, diarrhea, perspiration, or severe burns. Oliguria leading to anuria, cessation of urine flow, may result from any serious damage to the kidneys or from a decrease in the flow of blood to the kidneys. Two or three times more urine is excreted during the day than at night. An increase in the nocturnal excretion of urine is termed nocturia. Polyuria, an increase in daily urine volume, is often associated with diabetes mellitus and diabetes insipidus; however, it may also be artificially induced by the use of diuretics, caffeine, or alcohol, all of which suppress the secretion of antidiuretic hormone.

Diabetes mellitus and diabetes insipidus produce polyuria for different reasons, and analysis of the urine is an important step in the differential diagnosis. Diabetes mellitus is caused by a defect either in the production of insulin by the pancreas or in the function of insulin, resulting in an increased body glucose concentration. The excess glucose is not reabsorbed by the kidneys, necessitating the excretion of increased amounts of water to remove the dissolved glucose from the body. Although appearing to be dilute, a urine specimen from a patient with diabetes mellitus will have a high specific gravity due to the increased glucose content. Diabetes insipidus results from a decrease in the production or function of antidiuretic hormone; thus, the water necessary for adequate body hydration is not reabsorbed from the plasma filtrate. In this condition, the urine will be truly dilute and will have a low specific gravity. Fluid loss in both diseases is compensated for by increased ingestion of water, producing an even greater urine volume. Polyuria accompanied by increased fluid intake is often the first symptom of either disease.

SPECIMEN COLLECTION

The fact that a urine specimen is so readily available and easily collected often leads to laxity in the treatment of the specimen after it has been collected. Changes in urine composition take place not only in vivo, but also in vitro, thus necessitating correct handling procedures after the specimen is collected.

Three major rules of urine specimen handling actually apply to all specimens received in the laboratory:

1. The specimen must be collected in a clean, dry container. Disposable containers are becoming increasingly more popular both because they are cost-effective and because the chance of contamination due to improper washing has been eliminated. These disposable containers are available in a variety of sizes and shapes, including plastic bags with adhesive for the collection of pediatric specimens and large containers for 24-hour specimens.
2. The specimen containers must be properly labeled with the patient's name, the date and time of collection, and, when appropriate, additional information such as the hospital number and the doctor's name. Remember, several unlabeled urine specimens sitting on their respective requisition slips can easily be moved.
3. The specimen must be delivered to the laboratory promptly and tested within 1 hour. A specimen that cannot be delivered or tested within 2 hours should either be refrigerated or should have an appropriate chemical preservative added.

PRESERVATION

The most routinely used method of preservation is refrigeration, which is reliable in preventing bacterial decomposition of urine for an overnight period.[10] Refrigeration of the specimen can cause an increase in the specific gravity and the precipitation of amorphous phosphates and urates that may obscure the microscopic sediment analysis. However, allowing the specimen to return to room temperature prior to analysis will correct the specific gravity and may dissolve some of the amorphous urates. When a specimen must be transported over a long distance and refrigeration is not possible, chemical preservatives may be added. The ideal preservative should be bactericidal, inhibit urease, and preserve formed elements in the sediment. At the same time, it should not interfere with chemical tests.[3] Unfortunately, as can be seen in Table 1-2, the ideal preservative does not presently exist; therefore, it is important to choose a preservative that best suits the needs of the required analysis.

CHANGES IN UNPRESERVED URINE

Problems introduced by preservation can be considered minor if one considers the changes that take place in unpreserved urine. The following 10 changes may occur in a specimen allowed to remain unpreserved at room temperature for longer than 1 hour:

TABLE 1-2. Urine Preservatives

Preservative	Advantages	Disadvantages	Additional Information
Refrigeration	No interference with chemical tests	Raises specific gravity Precipitates amorphous phosphates and urates	Shown to prevent bacterial growth for at least 24 hours[10]
Thymol	Preserves glucose and sediments well	Interferes with acid precipitation tests for protein Large amounts will interfere with o-toluidine glucose tests	
Boric Acid	Preserves protein and formed elements well No interference with routine analyses other than pH	Large amounts are needed to inhibit bacterial growth Large amounts may cause crystal precipitation	Keeps pH at about 6.0 Interferes with drug and hormone analyses[8]
Formalin (Formaldehyde)	Excellent sediment preservative	Interferes with copper reduction tests for glucose	Containers for collection of specimens for Addis counts can be rinsed with formalin for better preservation of cells and casts
Chloroform	None	Sinks to the bottom of the specimen and interferes with sediment analysis Interferes with "falling drop" specific gravity	May cause cellular changes
Toluene	Does not interfere with routine chemical tests	Floats on the surface of specimens and clings to pipettes and testing materials	
Sodium Fluoride	Prevents glycolysis Good preservative for drug analyses[9]	Inhibits dipstick tests for glucose	Will not interfere with hexokinase tests for glucose Sodium benzoate instead of fluoride

TABLE 1-2. *Continued*

Preservative	Advantages	Disadvantages	Additional Information
			may be used for dipstick testing[7]
Hydrochloric Acid	Bactericidal	Destroys formed elements and precipitates solutes Unacceptable for routine analysis	May be dangerous to the patient[3]
Freezing	Preserves bilirubin and urobilinogen	Destroys formed elements Turbidity occurs upon thawing	Useful for nonroutine chemical analyses[6]
Commercial Preservative Tablets	Convenient when refrigeration is not possible Chemical concentration is controlled to minimize interference	May increase specific gravity[5] May contain one or more of the above chemical preservatives	Check tablet composition to determine possible effects on desired tests

1. increased **pH** from the breakdown of urea to ammonia by urease-producing bacteria
2. decreased **glucose** due to glycolysis and bacterial utilization
3. decreased **ketones** because of volatilization
4. decreased **bilirubin** from exposure to light
5. decreased **urobilinogen** by its oxidation to urobilin
6. increased **nitrite** due to bacterial reduction of nitrate
7. increased **bacteria**
8. increased **turbidity** caused by bacterial growth and possible precipitation of amorphous material
9. disintegration of **red blood cells** and **casts,** particularly in dilute alkaline urine
10. changes in **color** due to oxidation or reduction of metabolites.

These variations will be discussed again under the individual test procedures. At this point, it is important to realize that the results of a routine urinalysis can be seriously affected by improper preservation.

TYPES OF SPECIMENS

To obtain a specimen that is truly representative of a patient's metabolic state, it is often necessary to regulate certain aspects of specimen collection. These special conditions may include time of collection, length of collection, patient's dietary and medicinal intake, and method of collection. It is important to instruct patients when special collection procedures must be followed. Frequently encountered specimens are listed in Table 1-3.

TABLE 1-3. Types of Urine Specimens

Type of Specimen	Purpose
Random	Routine screening
First Morning	Routine screening Pregnancy tests Orthostatic protein
Fasting	Diabetic monitoring
2-Hour Postprandial	Diabetic monitoring Glucose testing
Glucose Tolerance Test (GTT)	Accompanies blood samples in glucose tolerance test
24-Hour (or timed)	Quantitative chemical tests
Catheterized	Bacterial culture
Midstream Clean-Catch	Routine screening Bacterial culture
Suprapubic Aspiration	Bladder urine for bacterial culture Cytology

RANDOM SPECIMEN

This is the most commonly received specimen due to the ease of collection and the lack of inconvenience to the patient. The random specimen is useful for routine screening tests to detect obvious abnormalities. However, it may also produce erroneous results due to dietary intake or physical activity just prior to the collection of the specimen. The patient will then be requested to collect additional specimens under more controlled conditions.

FIRST MORNING SPECIMEN

Although it may require the patient to make an additional trip to the laboratory, this is the ideal screening specimen. It is also essential for preventing false-negative pregnancy tests and for evaluating orthostatic proteinuria. The first morning specimen is a concentrated specimen, thereby assuring detection of substances that may not be present in a dilute random specimen. The patient should be instructed to collect the specimen immediately upon arising and to deliver it to the laboratory within 2 hours.

FASTING SPECIMEN

A fasting specimen differs from a first morning specimen by being the second voided specimen after a period of fasting. This specimen will not contain any metabolites from food ingested prior to the beginning of the fasting period.[4]

2-HOUR POSTPRANDIAL SPECIMEN

The patient is instructed to void shortly before consuming a routine meal and to collect a specimen 2 hours after eating. The specimen is tested for glucose, and the results are used primarily for monitoring insulin therapy in persons with diabetes mellitus. A more comprehensive evaluation of the patient's status can be obtained if the results of the 2-hour postprandial specimen are compared with those of a fasting specimen.

GLUCOSE TOLERANCE TEST (GTT) SPECIMENS

These specimens are collected to correspond with the blood samples drawn during a glucose tolerance test. The number of specimens varies with the length of the test. All tests will include fasting, $\frac{1}{2}$-hour, 1-hour, 2-hour, and 3-hour specimens, and possibly 4-, 5-, and 6-hour specimens. The urine is tested for glucose and ketones, and the results are reported with the blood test results as an aid to interpreting the patient's ability to metabolize a measured amount of glucose.

24-HOUR (OR TIMED) SPECIMEN

Often, it is necessary to measure the exact amount of a urine chemical rather than to just report its presence or absence. A carefully timed specimen must be used to produce accurate quantitative results. When the concentration of the substance to be measured varies with daily activities such as exercise, meals, and body metabolism, a 24-hour collection is required. If the concentration of the particular substance remains constant, the specimen may be collected over a shorter period of time. However, care must be taken to keep the patient adequately hydrated during short collection periods. Patients must be explicitly instructed on the procedure for collecting a timed specimen. To obtain an accurately timed specimen, it is necessary to begin the collection period with an empty bladder and to end the collection period with an empty bladder. The following instructions for collecting a 24-hour specimen can be applied to any timed collection.

> Day 1—7 AM: Patient voids and **discards** specimen. Patient **collects** all urine for the next 24 hours.
> Day 2—7 AM: Patient voids and **adds** this urine to the previously collected urine.

Upon its arrival in the laboratory, a 24-hour specimen must be thoroughly mixed and the volume accurately measured and recorded. If only an aliquot is needed for testing, the amount saved must be adequate to permit repeat or additional testing, if necessary. Consideration must also be given to the preservation of specimens collected over extended periods of time. The preservative chosen should be nontoxic to the patient and should not interfere with the tests to be performed. Appropriate collection information is included with test procedures and should be referred to before issuing a container and instructions to the patient. To ensure the accuracy of a 24-hour specimen, a known quantity of a nontoxic chemical marker, such as 4-aminobenzoic acid, may be given to the patient at the start of the collection period. The concentration of excreted marker in the specimen is measured to determine the completeness of the collection.[1]

CATHETERIZED SPECIMEN

This specimen is collected under sterile conditions by passing a hollow tube through the urethra into the bladder. The most commonly requested test on a catheterized specimen is a bacterial culture. If a routine urinalysis is also requested, the culture should be performed first to prevent contamination of the specimen.

A less frequently encountered type of catheterized specimen is used to measure functions in the individual kidneys. Specimens from the right and left kidneys are collected separately by passing catheters through the ureters of the respective kidneys.

MIDSTREAM CLEAN-CATCH SPECIMEN

As an alternative to the catheterized specimen, the midstream clean-catch specimen provides a safer, less traumatic method for obtaining urine for bacterial culture. This specimen also offers a more representative and less contaminated specimen for microscopic analysis than the routinely voided specimen. Patients must be provided with appropriate cleansing materials and a sterile container. They must also be thoroughly instructed in the methods for cleansing the genitalia and for collecting only the mid-stream portion of the urine.

SUPRAPUBIC ASPIRATION
Occasionally, urine may be collected by external introduction of a needle into the bladder. Since the bladder is sterile under normal conditions, this collection method provides a sample for bacterial culture that is completely free of extraneous contamination. The specimen can also be used for cytologic examination.

PEDIATRIC SPECIMENS
Collection of pediatric specimens can present a challenge. Soft, clear plastic bags with adhesive to attach to the genital area of both boys and girls are available for collecting routine specimens. Sterile specimens are obtained by catheterization or by suprapubic aspiration.

GLOSSARY
anuria. Complete stoppage of urine flow.

azotemia. Presence of increased nitrogenous waste products (primarily urea) in the blood.

catheter. Hollow tube for draining urine from the bladder or kidneys.

cystoscope. Instrument for examining the interior of the bladder and ureter.

diuresis. Passage of abnormally large amounts of urine.

diuretic. An agent that increases the formation of urine.

dysuria. Painful urination.

-emia. Relating to blood.

glycosuria (glucosuria). Glucose in the urine.

hematuria. Blood in the urine.

hypersthenuria. Urine with a specific gravity greater than the 1.010 specific gravity of the plasma filtrate.

hyposthenuria. Urine with a specific gravity less than the 1.010 specific gravity of the plasma filtrate.

isosthenuria. Urine with a specific gravity equal to the 1.010 specific gravity of the plasma filtrate.

ketonuria. Ketones in the urine.

nephritis. Inflammation of the kidney involving glomeruli, tubules, or interstitial tissue.

nephrology. The study of the structure and function of the kidney.

nocturia. Excessive urination during the night.

oliguria. Marked decrease in urine flow.

polyuria. Marked increase in urine flow.

proteinuria (albuminuria). Protein in the urine.

pyuria. Pus in the urine.

refractometer. Instrument used for indirectly determining specific gravity by refractive index.

renal. Pertaining to the kidney.

renal calculi. Kidney stones.

renal dialysis. Procedure used to remove waste products from the blood when kidneys are not functioning.

uremia. Presence of increased urea in the blood.

-uria. Relating to the urine.

urinalysis (complete or routine). The physical, chemical, and microscopic analysis of urine.

urinometer. Instrument used to directly measure the specific gravity of urine.

urologist. Physician specializing in the study of urology.

urology. Branch of medicine concerned with the male and female urinary tracts and the male genital tract.

ABBREVIATIONS

Abbreviation	Definition
ADH	Antidiuretic hormone
BJP	Bence Jones protein
BUN	Blood urea nitrogen
GTT	Glucose tolerance test
GU	Genitourinary
HCG	Human chorionic gonadotropin (pregnancy testing)
hpf	High-power field
IVP	Intravenous pyelogram (procedure performed in radiology using an opaque dye)
lpf	Low-power field
PKU	Phenylketonuria
2 hr pp or pc	Two hours after eating (postprandial or postcibal)
PSP	Phenolsulfonphthalein (dye used in renal function testing)
Q.C.	Quality control
qns	Quantity nonsufficient
RBC	red blood cell
Sp. Gr. or SG	Specific gravity
TNTC	Too numerous to count (e.g., WBC/hpf = TNTC)
UA	Routine urinalysis
WBC	White blood cell
WBC/hpf	Number of white blood cells seen per high-power field

REFERENCES

1. BINGHAM, S AND CUMMINGS, JH: *The use of 4-aminobenzoic acid as a marker to validate the completeness of 24 hour urine collections in man.* Clin Sci 64(6):629–635, 1984.
2. BRADLEY, B AND SCHUMANN, GB: *Examination of urine.* In HENRY, JB (ED): *Clinical Diagnosis and Management by Laboratory Methods.* WB Saunders, Philadelphia, 1979.
3. GRIFFITH, DP AND DUNN, D: *Collection and preservation of urine for biochemical analysis.* Invest Urol 15(6):459–461, 1978.
4. GUTHRIE, D, HINNEN, D, AND GUTHRIE, R: *Single-voided vs. double-voided urine testing.* Diabetes Care 2(3):269–271, 1979.
5. HERMAN, JR: *Urology: A View Through the Retrospectroscope.* Harper & Row, Hagerstown, Maryland, 1973.
6. LEACH, CS, RAMBAULT, PC, AND FISCHER, CL: *A comparative study of two methods of urine preservation.* Clin Biochem 8(2):108–117, 1975.
7. ONSTAD, J, HANCOCK, D, AND WOLF, P: *Inhibitory effect of fluoride on glucose tests with glucose oxidase strips.* Clin Chem 21:898–899, 1975.
8. PORTER, IA AND BRODIE, J: *Boric acid preservation of urine samples.* Br Med J 2:353–355, 1969.
9. ROCKERBIE, RA AND CAMPBELL, DJ: *Effect of specimen storage and preservation on toxicological analysis of urine.* Clin Biochem 11(3):77–81, 1978.
10. RYAN, WL AND MILLS, RD: *Bacterial multiplication in urine during refrigeration.* Am J Med Technol 29:175–177, 1963.

STUDY QUESTIONS (Choose one best answer)

1. The primary chemical constituents of normal urine are:

   a. water, protein, and sodium
   b. water, urea, and protein
   c. water, urea, and chloride
   d. water, urea, and bilirubin

2. A person exhibiting oliguria would have a daily urine volume of:

   a. 200–600 ml
   b. 600–1000 ml
   c. 1000–1500 ml
   d. over 1500 ml

3. In forensic pathology, it is sometimes necessary to determine if a specimen is actually urine. To do this, you would measure the content of:

   a. chloride and sodium
   b. urea and creatinine
   c. uric acid and amino acids
   d. protein and amino acids

4. Urine from patients with diabetes mellitus has:

   a. decreased volume and decreased specific gravity
   b. decreased volume and increased specific gravity
   c. increased volume and decreased specific gravity
   d. increased volume and increased specific gravity

5. A specimen containing precipitated amorphous phosphates may have been preserved using:

   a. boric acid
   b. chloroform
   c. formalin
   d. refrigeration

6. For the best preservation of urinary sediments, the preservatives of choice are:

   a. boric and hydrochloric acids
   b. thymol and formalin
   c. formalin and freezing
   d. chloroform and refrigeration

7. An unpreserved specimen collected at 8 AM and remaining at room temperature until the afternoon shift arrives can be expected to have:

   1. decreased glucose and ketones
   2. increased bacteria and nitrite
   3. decreased pH and turbidity
   4. decreased cellular elements
   a. 1, 2, and 3
   b. 1, 2, and 4
   c. 1 and 2 only
   d. 4 only

8. Red blood cells will disintegrate more rapidly in urine that is:

   a. concentrated and acidic
   b. concentrated and alkaline
   c. dilute and acidic
   d. dilute and alkaline

9. Quantitative urine tests are most accurately performed on:

   a. first morning specimens
   b. timed specimens
   c. midstream clean-catch specimens
   d. suprapubic aspirations

10. A first morning urine is the specimen of choice for routine urinalysis because:

    a. it has a high volume
    b. it is produced while the body is in a resting state
    c. it is more concentrated, resulting in better detection of abnormalities
    d. it is more dilute, preventing false-positive reactions

11. Cessation of urine flow is termed:

    a. azotemia
    b. dysuria
    c. diuresis
    d. anuria

12. Persons taking diuretics can be expected to produce:

    a. proteinuria
    b. polyuria
    c. pyuria
    d. oliguria

13. Mary Johnson brings a urine specimen to the laboratory with a requisition for a glucose determination. The test is negative. Mary's doctor questions this result because she has a family history of diabetes mellitus and is experiencing mild clinical symptoms of the disease. What two possibilities regarding the urine specimen could account for a possible false-negative reaction with Mary's glucose test?

14. How could a specimen be obtained that would more accurately reflect Mary's glucose metabolism?

2
FUNCTION AND DISEASES OF THE KIDNEY

INSTRUCTIONAL OBJECTIVES

Upon completion of this chapter, readers will be able to:

1. discuss the physiologic mechanisms of glomerular filtration, tubular reabsorption, tubular secretion, and renal blood flow

2. identify the laboratory procedures used to evaluate these four renal functions

3. differentiate between exogenous and endogenous procedures

4. explain why creatinine is the substance of choice for testing glomerular filtration rates

5. given hypothetical laboratory data, calculate a creatinine clearance and determine if the result is normal

6. describe the Fishberg and Mosenthal concentration tests, including specimen collection, testing, and normal results

7. define osmolarity and discuss its relationship to urine concentration

8. describe the basic principles of clinical osmometers

9. given hypothetical laboratory data, calculate a free water clearance and interpret the result

10. discuss the PSP test with regard to specimen collection, chemical testing, and physiologic principle

11. given hypothetical laboratory data, calculate a PAH clearance and relate this result to renal blood flow

12. describe the relationship of ammonia to urinary titratable acidity and to the production of an acidic urine

13. state the primary cause of acute glomerulonephritis and describe the major urinalysis findings

14. briefly discuss the chronic forms of glomerular disease, the nephrotic syndrome, and renal failure, including the renal functions affected and significant urinalysis results

15. describe the urine sediment in pyelonephritis

This chapter presents a review of nephron anatomy and physiology and its relationship to urinalysis and renal function testing, followed by a section on laboratory assessment of renal function and a discussion of the major renal diseases.

RENAL PHYSIOLOGY

Each kidney contains approximately 1 to 1.5 million nephrons. Figure 2-1 shows the relationship of the nephron to the kidney and excretory system, and Figure 2-2 provides a composite view of the nephron. The kidneys' ability to selectively clear waste products from the blood and at the same time to maintain the essential water and electrolyte balances in the body is controlled in the nephron by the following renal functions: renal blood flow, glomerular filtration, tubular reabsorption, and tubular secretion. The physiology, laboratory testing, and associated pathology of these four functions are discussed in this chapter.

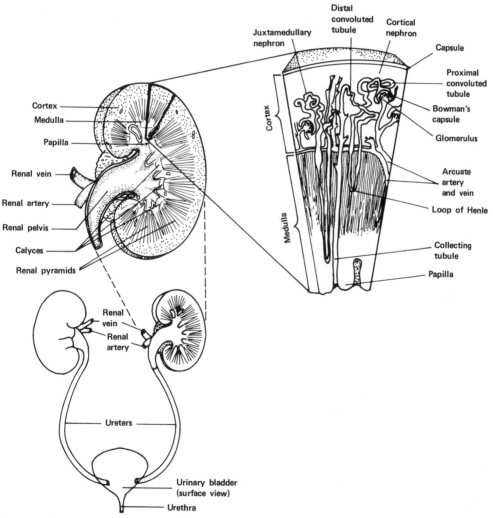

FIGURE 2-1. The relationship of the nephron to the kidney and excretory system. (Adapted from Spence, A. and Mason, E.: *Human Anatomy and Physiology*. Benjamin/Cummings Publishing, Menlo Park, California, 1983; and Previte, J. J.: *Human Physiology*. McGraw-Hill, New York, 1983.)

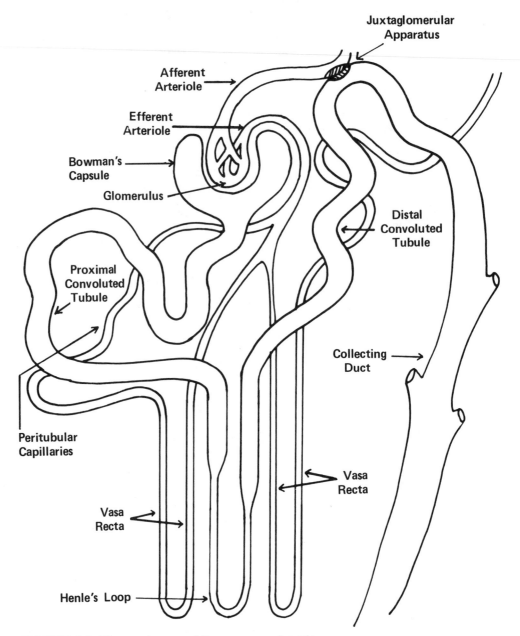

FIGURE 2-2. The nephron and its component parts.

RENAL BLOOD FLOW

Blood is supplied to the kidney by the renal artery and enters the nephron through the afferent arteriole. It flows through the glomerulus and into the efferent arteriole. The ability of these arterioles to vary in size helps to create the hydrostatic pressure differential important for glomerular filtration and to maintain consistency of glomerular capillary pressure and renal blood flow within the glomerulus. Notice the smaller size of the efferent arteriole in Figure 2-2. This produces an increase in the glomerular capillary pressure. Before returning to the renal vein, the blood from the efferent arteriole enters the peritubular capillaries and the vasa recta and flows slowly through the cortex and medulla of the kidney in close proximity to the tubules. The peritubular capillaries surround the proximal and distal convoluted tubules, providing for the immediate reabsorption of essential substances from the fluid in the proximal convoluted tubule and final adjustment of the urinary composition in the distal convoluted tubule. The vasa recta are located adjacent to the ascending and descending loops of Henle, and it is in this area that the major exchanges of water and salts take place.

Based on an average body size of 1.73 square meters of surface, the total renal blood flow is approximately 1200 ml per minute, and the total renal plasma flow ranges from 600 to 700 ml per minute. Normal values for renal blood flow and renal function tests are dependent on body size. When dealing with sizes that vary greatly from the average 1.73 square meters of surface, a correction must be calculated to determine if the observed measurements represent normal function. This calculation is covered in the discussion on tests for glomerular filtration rate. Variations in normal values have also been published for different age groups and should be taken into consideration when evaluating renal function studies.

GLOMERULAR FILTRATION

Blood from the afferent arteriole enters the glomerulus within Bowman's capsule. The glomerulus consists of a coil of approximately eight capillary lobes referred to collectively as the capillary tuft. Although the glomerulus serves as a nonselective filter of plasma substances with molecular weights of less than 70,000, several factors influence the actual filtration process. These include the cellular structure of the capillary walls and Bowman's capsule, hydrostatic and oncotic pressures, and the feedback mechanisms of the renin-angiotensin system and aldosterone. Figure 2-3 provides a diagrammatic view of the glomerular areas influenced by these factors.

Plasma filtrate must pass through three cellular layers: the capillary wall membrane, the basement membrane (basal lamina), and the visceral epithelium of Bowman's capsule. The endothelial cells of the capillary wall differ from those in other capillaries by containing pores and are referred to as fenestrated. The pores increase capillary permeability but do not allow the passage of large molecules and blood cells. Further restriction of large molecules occurs as the filtrate passes through the basement membrane and the thin membranes covering the filtration slits formed by the intertwining foot processes of the visceral epithelial podocytes (see Fig. 2-3).

As mentioned earlier, filtration is enhanced by the presence of hydrostatic pressure created by the smaller size of the efferent arteriole. This pressure is necessary to overcome the opposition of pressures from the fluid within Bowman's capsule and the colloidal pressure of plasma proteins. By increasing or decreasing the size of the afferent arteriole, an autoregulatory mechanism within the kidney maintains the glomerular blood pressure at a relatively constant rate regardless of fluctuations in systemic blood pressure. Dilation of the afferent arterioles when blood pressure drops prevents a marked decrease in blood flowing through the kidney, thus preventing a rise in the blood level of toxic waste products.

Additional influence on the flow of blood through the kidney is provided by the renin-angiotensin system and aldosterone, which are activated in response to changes in blood flow to the kidney sensed by the macula densa in the juxtamedullary apparatus (see Fig. 2-2). The hormone aldosterone is secreted by the adrenal cortex and increases the reabsorption of sodium from the glomerular filtrate. Renin, an enzyme that is produced in the kidney when blood pressure levels decline, causes the production of angiotensin II, a potent vasoconstrictor. Renin also stimulates the production of aldosterone, which increases the reabsorption of sodium. This results in water retention, which increases extracellular fluid volume and intravascular pressure. As systemic pressure increases, production of renin is decreased, thus producing a decrease in angiotensin and aldosterone levels.

As a result of the above glomerular mechanisms, every minute approximately 120 ml of water containing low molecular weight substances are filtered through the two million glomeruli. Because this filtration is nonselective, the only difference between the compositions of the filtrate and the plasma is the absence of plasma protein, any protein-bound substances, and cells. Analysis of the fluid as it leaves the glomerulus

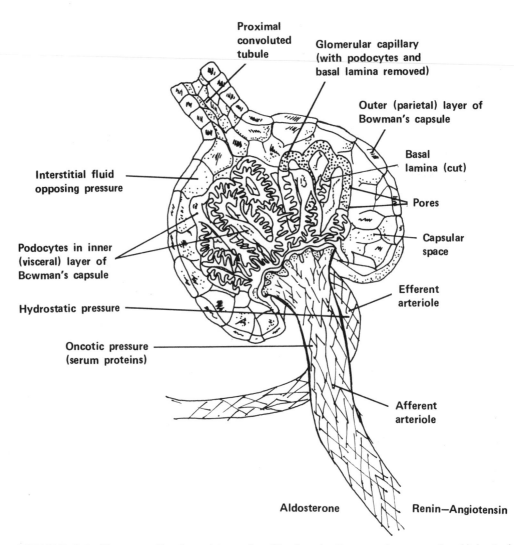

Proximal
convoluted
tubule

Glomerular capillary
(with podocytes and
basal lamina removed)

Outer (parietal) layer of
Bowman's capsule

Basal
lamina (cut)

Pores

Capsular
space

Interstitial fluid
opposing pressure

Podocytes in inner
(visceral) layer of
Bowman's capsule

Hydrostatic pressure

Oncotic pressure
(serum proteins)

Efferent
arteriole

Afferent
arteriole

Aldosterone

Renin—Angiotensin

FIGURE 2-3. Factors affecting glomerular filtration in the renal corpuscle. (Adapted from Spence, A. and Mason, E.: *Human Anatomy and Physiology.* Benjamin/Cummings Publishing, Menlo Park, California, 1983.)

shows the filtrate to have a specific gravity of 1.010 and confirms that it is chemically an ultrafiltrate of plasma. This information provides a useful baseline for evaluating the renal mechanisms involved in converting the plasma ultrafiltrate into the final urinary product.

TUBULAR REABSORPTION

It is obvious that the body cannot lose 120 ml of water containing essential substances every minute. Therefore, when the plasma ultrafiltrate enters the proximal convoluted tubule, the kidney, through cellular transport mechanisms, begins reabsorbing these essential substances and water. Table 2-1 provides a comparison of the chemical content of plasma, glomerular filtrate, and urine. The cellular mechanisms involved in tubular reabsorption are termed active and passive transport. For active transport to occur, the substance to be reabsorbed must combine with a carrier protein contained in the membranes of the cells lining the tubules. The electrochemical energy created by this interaction transfers the substance across the cell membranes and back into the blood stream. Active transport is responsible for the reabsorption of glucose, amino

TABLE 2-1. Comparison of Chemical Content of Plasma, Glomerular Filtrate, and Urine*

Substance	Concentrations (mg/100 ml)		
	Plasma	Glomerular Filtrate	Urine
Glucose	100	100	0
Urea	26	26	1820
Uric acid	4	4	50
Creatinine	1	1	190

Substance	Concentrations (mEq/liter)		
	Plasma	Glomerular Filtrate	Urine
Sodium (Na^+)	142	142	125
Potassium (K^+)	5	5	60
Calcium (Ca^{2+})	4	4	5
Magnesium (Mg^{2+})	3	3	15
Chlorine (Cl^-)	103	103	130
Bicarbonate (HCO_3^-)	27	27	14
Sulfate (SO_4^2)	1	1	33
Phosphate (PO_4^{3-})	2	2	40

*From Creager, JG: *Human Anatomy and Physiology.* Wadsworth Publishing, Belmont, California, 1983, p. 660, with permission.

acids, and salts in the proximal convoluted tubule, and the reabsorption of sodium in the ascending loop of Henle and the distal convoluted tubule. Passive transport is the movement of molecules across a membrane as a result of differences in their concentration or electrical potential on opposite sides of the membrane. These physical differences are called gradients. Passive reabsorption of water takes place in all parts of the nephron except the ascending loop of Henle, the walls of which are impermeable to water. Urea is also passively reabsorbed in the proximal convoluted tubule and the ascending loop of Henle.

Active transport, like passive transport, can also be influenced by the plasma concentration of the substance being transported. When the plasma concentration of a substance that is usually completely reabsorbed reaches an abnormally high level, active transport stops, and the substance then begins appearing in the urine. The plasma concentration at which active transport ceases is the "renal threshold." For glucose, the renal threshold is 160 to 180 mg per dl, and glycosuria occurs when the plasma concentration reaches this level. Substances that are completely reabsorbed until the renal threshold is reached (such as glucose) are termed high-threshold substances.

Active transport in the proximal convoluted tubule is accompanied by the passive reabsorption of water. Therefore, as can be seen in Figure 2-4, the fluid leaving the proximal convoluted tubule still maintains the same concentration (osmolality) as the ultrafiltrate. Actual concentration of the filtrate takes place primarily in the descending and ascending loops of Henle, where the filtrate is exposed to the high osmotic gradient

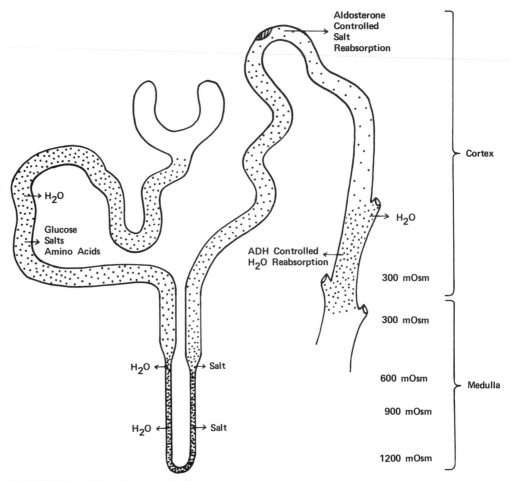

FIGURE 2-4. Renal concentration.

(salt concentration) of the renal medulla. Water is removed by osmosis in the descending loop of Henle, and sodium and chloride molecules are reabsorbed by active transport in the ascending loop of Henle. Excessive reabsorption of water as the filtrate passes through the highly concentrated medulla is prevented by the water-impermeable walls of the ascending loop of Henle. This selective reabsorption process in the loops of Henle is called the countercurrent mechanism, which not only concentrates the filtrate, but also maintains the osmotic gradient in the medulla.[15] In other words, the sodium that is removed from the fluid in the ascending loop prevents dilution of the medullary interstitium by the water diffusing from the descending loop.

Reabsorption continues in the distal convoluted tubule and the collecting duct, but it is now under the control of the hormones aldosterone and vasopressin (antidiuretic hormone [ADH]). In response to body requirements for sodium, aldosterone regulates its reabsorption in the distal convoluted tubule. Likewise, ADH can control body hydration by rendering the walls of the distal convoluted tubules and the collecting duct permeable or impermeable to water. Under conditions of dehydration, the presence of a high level of ADH increases the permeability, resulting in increased reabsorption of water and a low urine volume. Therefore, the electrolyte balance in the body is the final determinant of urine volume and concentration.

TUBULAR SECRETION

In contrast to tubular reabsorption, in which substances are removed from the glomerular filtrate and returned to the blood, tubular secretion involves the passage of sub-

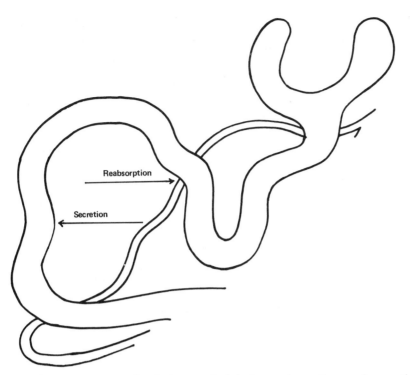

FIGURE 2-5. The movement of substances in tubular reabsorption and secretion.

stances from the blood in the peritubular capillaries to the tubular filtrate (Fig. 2-5). Tubular secretion serves two major functions: elimination of waste products not filtered by the glomerulus, and regulation of the acid-base balance in the body through the secretion of hydrogen ions. Many foreign substances, such as medications, cannot be filtered by the glomerulus because they are bound to plasma proteins. However, when these protein-bound substances enter the peritubular capillaries, they develop a strong affinity for the tubular cells and dissociate from their carrier proteins, which results in

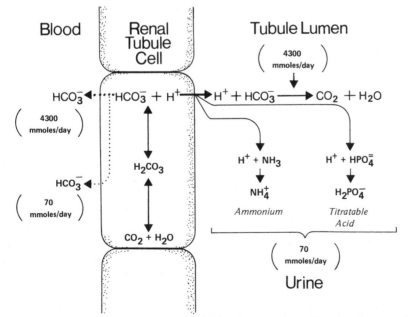

FIGURE 2-6. Schematic representation of bicarbonate handling by the renal tubule. (From Forland, M,[8] p. 30, with permission.)

their transportation into the filtrate by the tubular cells. The major site for removal of these nonfiltered substances is the proximal convoluted tubule.

To maintain the normal blood pH of 7.4, it is necessary to buffer and eliminate the excess acid formed from dietary intake and metabolism. Much of the excess acid is eliminated through the lungs in the form of carbon dioxide. However, the buffering capacity of the blood is dependent on bicarbonate ions, which are readily filtered by the glomerulus and must be expediently returned to the blood to maintain proper pH. As shown in Figure 2-6, secretion of hydrogen ions in the proximal convoluted tubule facilitates this process. Aided by the enzyme carbonic anhydrase, the filtered bicarbonate combines with the secreted hydrogen ion to form carbonic acid, which readily dissociates into carbon dioxide and water. Carbon dioxide easily diffuses back into the tubular cells to combine with water to form carbonic acid, which again dissociates into bicarbonate ion and hydrogen ion. The bicarbonate is reabsorbed into the blood, and the hydrogen is secreted back into the filtrate to combine with another filtered bicarbonate ion. This process provides almost 100 percent reabsorption of filtered bicarbonate. Additional hydrogen ions combine with either filtered phosphates and are excreted as titratable acid, or with ammonia produced and secreted by the distal convoluted tubule. The combining of excess hydrogen ions with ammonia ensures their excretion because the resulting ammonium ion will not be reabsorbed as would the free hydrogen ion.

RENAL FUNCTION TESTS

As can be seen from the brief review of renal physiology, there are many metabolic functions and chemical interactions to be evaluated through laboratory tests of renal function. Figure 2-7 relates the parts of the nephron to the laboratory tests used to assess their function.

GLOMERULAR FILTRATION TESTS

The standard test used to measure the filtering capacity of the glomeruli is the clearance test. As its name implies, a clearance test measures the rate at which the kidneys are able to remove (clear) a filterable substance from the blood. To ensure that glomerular filtration is being accurately measured, the substance analyzed must be one that is neither reabsorbed nor secreted by the tubules. Furthermore, the stability of the substance in urine during a possible 24-hour collection period, the consistency of the plasma level, the substance's availability to the body, and the ease of chemical analysis of the substance are also factors that must be taken into consideration in the selection of a clearance test substance.

CLEARANCE TESTS

The earliest glomerular filtration tests measured urea because of its presence in all urine specimens and the existence of proven methods of chemical analysis. Since approximately 40 percent of the filtered urea is reabsorbed, normal values were adjusted to reflect the reabsorption, and patients were hydrated to produce a urine flow of 2 ml per minute to ensure that no more than 40 percent of the urea was reabsorbed. At the present time, the use of urea as a test substance for glomerular filtration has been almost entirely replaced by the measurement of either creatinine, inulin, or radioisotopes. With only minor exceptions, both creatinine and inulin meet the necessary criteria for a clearance test substance. Inulin, a polymer of fructose, is an extremely stable substance that is not reabsorbed or secreted by the tubules. However, it is not a normal body constituent and must be infused at a constant rate throughout the testing period. A test that requires an infused substance is termed an exogenous procedure and is seldom the method of choice if a suitable test substance is already present in the body (endogenous procedure). Therefore, inulin has not been routinely used for

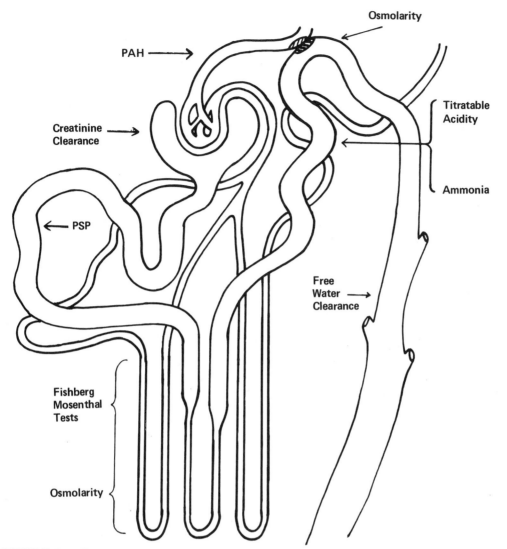

FIGURE 2-7. The relationship of nephron areas to renal function tests.

glomerular filtration testing, although the recent development of simplified inulin infusion procedures and the use of radioisotopes to measure glomerular filtration rate may increase the use of these exogenous substances.[22,4] Currently, routine laboratory measurements of glomerular filtration rate employ creatinine as the test substance. Creatinine, a waste product of muscle metabolism that is normally found at a constant level in the blood, provides the laboratory with an endogenous procedure for evaluating glomerular function. The use of creatinine has several disadvantages not found with inulin, including:

1. Some creatinine may be secreted by the tubules when blood levels are high, as occurs in advanced renal disease.
2. Serum chromogens that are often present in advanced renal disease may react in the chemical analysis. However, these interfering substances can be removed prior to analysis.
3. Urinary creatinine will be broken down by bacteria if specimens are kept at room temperature for extended periods of time.[19]
4. A heavy meat diet consumed during collection of a 24-hour urine specimen may influence the results if the plasma specimen is drawn prior to the collection period.[14]

5. Measurement of creatinine clearance is not a reliable indicator in patients suffering from muscle-wasting diseases.[21]

However, with careful laboratory technique and appropriate clinical correlation, a reliable endogenous measurement of the glomerular filtration rate can be obtained using the creatinine clearance method.

CALCULATIONS

By far the greatest source of error in any clearance procedure is the use of improperly timed urine specimens. The importance of using an accurately timed specimen, as described in Chapter 1, will become evident as we now discuss the calculations involved in converting isolated laboratory measurements to glomerular filtration rate. The glomerular filtration rate is reported in milliliters per minute; therefore, it is necessary to determine the number of milliliters of plasma from which the clearance substance (creatinine) is completely removed during a 1-minute period. To calculate this information, one must know: (V) urine volume in ml per minute, (U) urine creatinine concentration in mg per dl, and (P) plasma creatinine concentration in mg per dl.

The urine volume is calculated by dividing the number of milliliters in the specimen by the number of minutes used to collect the specimen.

Example: Calculate the urine volume for a 2-hour specimen measuring 240 milliliters.

$$2 \text{ hours} \times 60 \text{ minutes} = 120 \text{ minutes}$$

$$\frac{240 \text{ ml}}{120 \text{ min}} = 2 \text{ ml/min} \qquad V = 2 \text{ ml/min}$$

The plasma and urine concentrations are determined by chemical testing. The standard formula used to calculate the milliliters of plasma cleared per minute (C) is $C = \dfrac{UV}{P}$.

This formula is derived as follows: the milliliters of plasma cleared per minute (C) times the milligrams per deciliter of plasma creatinine (P) must equal the milligrams per deciliter of urine creatinine (U) times the urine volume in milliliters per minute (V), because all of the filtered creatinine will appear in the urine. Therefore, $CP = UV$ and $C = \dfrac{UV}{P}$.

Example: Using (U) urine creatinine of 120 mg/dl, (P) plasma creatinine of 1.0 mg/dl, and (V) urine volume of 60 ml obtained from a 1-hour specimen, calculate (C) the glomerular filtration rate (creatinine clearance).

$$V = \frac{60 \text{ ml}}{60 \text{ min}} = 1 \text{ ml/min}$$

$$C = \frac{120 \text{ mg/dl (U)} \times 1 \text{ ml/min (V)}}{1.0 \text{ mg/dl (P)}} = 120 \text{ ml/min}$$

By analyzing this calculation and Figure 2-8, we can see that at a 1 mg per dl concentration, each milliliter of plasma contains 0.01 mg creatinine. Therefore, to arrive at a urine concentration of 120 mg per dl (1.2 mg per ml), it would be necessary to clear 120 ml of plasma. Notice also that although the filtrate volume is reduced, the amount of creatinine in the filtrate does not change.

Knowing that in the average person (1.73 square meter body surface) the approximate amount of plasma filtrate produced per minute is 120 ml, it is not surprising that normal creatinine clearance values approach 120 ml per min (men, 107 to 139 ml per min; women, 87 to 107 ml per min). The normal plasma creatinine is 0.5 to 1.5 mg per

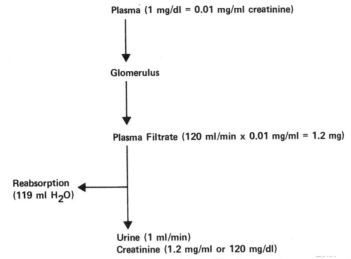

Plasma (1 mg/dl = 0.01 mg/ml creatinine)

Glomerulus

Plasma Filtrate (120 ml/min x 0.01 mg/ml = 1.2 mg)

Reabsorption
(119 ml H₂O)

Urine (1 ml/min)
Creatinine (1.2 mg/ml or 120 mg/dl)

FIGURE 2-8. A diagram representing creatinine filtration and excretion.

dl. These normal values take into account variations in size and muscle mass. However, values are considerably lower in older people, and an adjustment may also have to be made to the calculation when dealing with body sizes that deviate greatly from 1.73 square meters of surface, such as in children. To adjust a clearance due to body size, the formula is: $C = \dfrac{UV}{P} \times \dfrac{1.73}{A}$, with A being the actual body size in square meters of surface. The actual body size may be calculated as: $\log A = (0.425 \times \log \text{weight}) + (0.725 \times \log \text{height}) - 2.144$, or it may be obtained from the nomogram shown in Figure 2-9.

CLINICAL SIGNIFICANCE

When interpreting the results of a creatinine clearance test, one must keep in mind that the glomerular filtration rate is determined not only by the number of functioning nephrons, but also by the functional capacity of these nephrons. In other words, even though one half of the available nephrons may be nonfunctional, a change in the glomerular filtration rate will not occur if the remaining nephrons double their filtering capacity. This is evidenced by those persons who lead normal lives with only one kidney. Therefore, although the creatinine clearance is a frequently requested laboratory procedure, its value does not lie in the detection of early renal disease. It is used, instead, to determine the extent of nephron damage in known cases of renal disease, to monitor the effectiveness of treatment designed to prevent further nephron damage, and to determine the feasibility of administering drugs, such as antibiotics, that can build up to dangerous blood levels if the glomerular filtration rate is markedly reduced.

TUBULAR REABSORPTION TESTS

Whereas measurement of the glomerular filtration rate is not a useful indication of early renal disease, the loss of tubular reabsorption ability is often the first function affected in renal disease. This is not surprising when one considers the complexity of the tubular reabsorption process.

Tests to determine the ability of the tubules to reabsorb the essential salts and water that have been nonselectively filtered by the glomerulus are collectively termed concentration tests. As mentioned earlier, the ultrafiltrate that enters the tubules has a specific gravity of 1.010; therefore, after reabsorption one would expect the final urine product to be more concentrated. However, from our experience in performing routine urinalysis, we know that many specimens do not have a specific gravity higher than

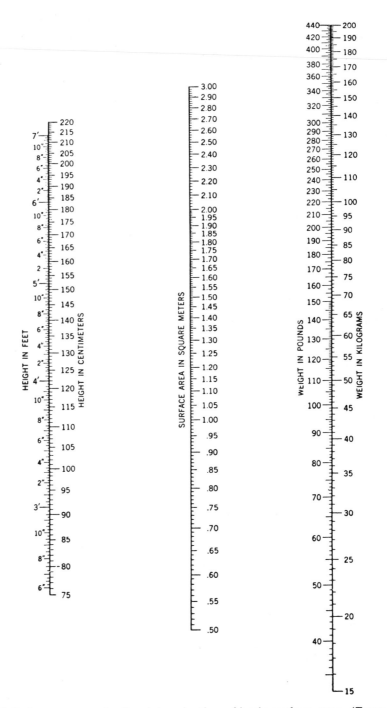

FIGURE 2-9. A nomogram for the determination of body surface area. (From Boothby, WM, and Sandiford, RB: *Nomogram for determination of body surface area.* N Engl J Med 185:337, 1921, with permission.)

1.010; yet, there is no renal disease present. This is because urine concentration is largely determined by the body's state of hydration, and the normal kidney will only reabsorb the amount of water necessary to preserve an adequate supply of body water.

As can be seen in Figure 2-10, both specimens contain the same amount of solute; however, the urine density (specific gravity) of Patient A will be higher. Therefore, control of fluid intake must be incorporated into laboratory tests that measure the concentrating ability of the kidney. Various methods are available to provide water depri-

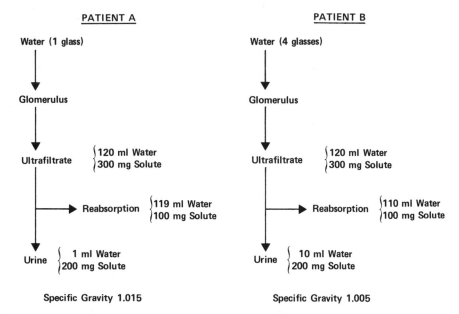

FIGURE 2-10. The effect of hydration on specific gravity.

vation and controlled specimens for analysis. Two well-known procedures are the Fishberg and Mosenthal tests.

FISHBERG TEST

In the Fishberg concentration test, the patient eats a normal breakfast and then consumes no more fluid until 8 AM the next morning. At that time, the patient collects a urine specimen, then remains in bed for 1 hour, collects another specimen, resumes normal activity for 1 hour, then collects a third specimen. The specific gravity of at least one of these specimens should be 1.026 or higher. A simplified version of the Fishberg procedure that is routinely used in many laboratories requires the patient to restrict fluids either with or immediately following the evening meal and then to collect specimens at 7 AM, 8 AM, and 9 AM the following morning. Each specimen is tested for specific gravity, and at least one specimen should measure 1.022 or higher. With both of these procedures, the first specimen voided may not have the highest specific gravity, as nocturnal diuresis in some patients produces a diluted first specimen.

MOSENTHAL TEST

The Mosenthal test allows the patient to maintain a normal diet and fluid intake; however, urine is collected over a 24-hour period. After emptying the bladder at 8 AM, the patient is instructed to collect all urine passed between 8 AM and 8 PM in one container and to collect all urine passed between 8 PM and 8 AM in a second container. In the laboratory, both specimens are measured and tested for specific gravity. Persons with normal concentrating ability will produce a day specimen (8 AM to 8 PM) with a higher volume and lower specific gravity than the night specimen (8 PM to 8 AM).

OSMOLARITY

Although the simplicity of the specific gravity measurements employed in the Fishberg and Mosenthal tests is convenient for routine clinical use, a more accurate evaluation of renal concentrating ability can be obtained by measuring serum and urine osmolarity. Specific gravity (measured by urinometry or refractometry) depends on the number of particles present in a solution and the density of these particles; whereas osmolarity is affected only by the number of particles present. When evaluating renal concentrating ability, the substances of interest are small molecules, primarily sodium (molecular weight, 23) and chloride (molecular weight, 35.5). However, urea (molecular weight, 60), which is of no importance to this evaluation, will contribute more to the specific gravity than the sodium and chloride molecules. Because all three of these molecules contribute equally to the osmolarity of the specimen, a more representative measure of renal concentrating ability can be obtained by measuring osmolarity. The correlation between specific gravity measured by reagent strips and osmolarity is currently being investigated.[9]

An osmole is defined as one gram molecular weight of a substance divided by the number of particles into which it dissociates.[5] A nonionizing substance such as glucose (molecular weight, 180) would contain 180 grams per osmole; whereas NaCl (molecular weight, 58.5), if completely dissociated, would contain 29.25 grams per osmole. Just as we have the terms molality and molarity, we have osmolality and osmolarity. An osmolal solution of glucose would have 180 grams of glucose dissolved in one kilogram of solvent, and an osmolar solution would have 180 grams of glucose dissolved in one liter of solvent. In the clinical laboratory, the terms are used interchangeably, since the difference under normal temperature conditions with water as the solvent is minimal. The unit of measure used in the clinical laboratory is the milliosmole (mOsm) because it is not practical, when dealing with body fluids, to use a measurement as large as the osmole (23 grams of sodium per liter or kilogram). The osmolarity of a solution can be determined by measuring a property that is mathematically related to the number of particles in the solution (colligative property) and comparing this value to the value obtained from the pure solvent. Solute dissolved in solvent causes the following changes in colligative properties: lower freezing point, higher boiling point, increased osmotic pressure, and lower vapor pressure.

Since water is the solvent in both urine and plasma, it is possible to determine the number of particles present in a sample by comparing a colligative property value of the sample to that of pure water. Clinical laboratory instruments are available to measure freezing point depression and vapor pressure depression.

CLINICAL OSMOMETERS

Measurement of freezing point depression was the first principle incorporated into clinical osmometers, and many instruments employing this technique are available. These osmometers determine the freezing point of a solution by supercooling a measured amount of sample to approximately $-7°C$. The supercooled sample is then vibrated to produce crystallization of water in the solution. The heat of fusion produced by the crystallizing water temporarily raises the temperature of the solution to its freezing point. A temperature-sensitive probe measures this temperature rise, and this information is transferred by means of a Wheatstone bridge to a galvanometer and converted into milliosmoles.[25] Conversion is made possible by the fact that 1 mole (1000 mOsm) of a nonionizing substance dissolved in 1 kilogram of water is known to lower the freezing point $1.86°C$. Therefore, by comparing the freezing point depression of a solution containing ionizing and nonionizing substances to the $-1.86°C$ depression of a solution of nonionizing substance, the number of milliosmoles in the mixed solution can be determined.

Example: One mole of NaCl dissolved in one kilogram of water depresses the freezing point $-3.46°C$. Calculate the osmolarity of the solution.

$$\frac{1000 \text{ mOsm}}{-1.86} = \frac{X \text{ mOsm}}{-3.46}$$

$$-1.86X = -3.46 \times 1000$$

$$X = 1860 \text{ mOsm}$$

Clinical osmometers use solutions of NaCl as their reference standards because a solution of partially ionized substances is more representative of urine and plasma composition. Standards of both low and high concentration can be prepared in the manner shown above. The newest addition to clinical osmometry is called the vapor pressure osmometer. However, the actual measurement performed is the dew point (temperature at which water vapor condenses to a liquid). The depression of dew-point temperature by solute parallels the decrease in vapor pressure, thereby providing a measure of this colligative property. When a sample is introduced into the sealed chamber of a vapor pressure osmometer, the dew-point temperature is measured, compared with that of an NaCl standard, and converted into milliosmoles. The vapor pressure osmometer utilizes microsamples of less than 0.01 ml; therefore, care must be taken to prevent any evaporation of the sample prior to testing.[16]

CLINICAL SIGNIFICANCE

Factors that should be taken into consideration because of their influence on true osmolarity readings include lipemic serum and the presence of lactic acid or volatile substances, such as ethanol, in the specimen. In lipemic serum, the displacement of serum water by insoluble lipids produces erroneous results with both vapor pressure and freezing point osmometers. Falsely elevated values due to the formation of lactic acid will also occur with both methods if serum samples are not separated or refrigerated within 20 minutes.[18] Vapor pressure osmometers will not detect the presence of volatile substances, since they become part of the solvent phase; however, measurements performed on similar specimens using freezing point osmometers will be elevated. Weisberg[25] recommends the use of cryoscopic osmolarity testing to rapidly evaluate comatose patients for the presence of alcohol. Currently, clinical uses of osmolarity include initial evaluation of renal concentrating ability, monitoring the course of renal disease, monitoring fluid and electrolyte therapy, establishing the differential diagnosis of hypernatremia and hyponatremia and polyuria, and evaluating the secretion of and renal response to ADH.[20].

Normal serum osmolarity values are between 275 and 300 mOsm. Normal values for urine osmolarity are difficult to establish, since factors such as diet and exercise can greatly influence the urine concentration and values can range between 50 and 1400 mOsm.[19] Therefore, it is often necessary to measure both serum and urine osmolarity and to evaluate the ratio obtained from the two readings. Under normal random conditions, the ratio of urine to serum osmolarity should be at least 1:1; after controlled fluid intake, it should reach 3:1. Determination of the urine-to-serum osmolarity ratio, in conjunction with procedures such as controlled fluid intake and injection of ADH, is used to differentiate the several types of diabetes insipidus, to aid in the identification of tumors that produce ADH-like substances, and to determine the underlying causes of apparent renal pathology.[2]

FREE WATER CLEARANCE

When dealing with difficult diagnostic problems, it may become necessary to further expand the urine-to-serum osmolarity ratio by performing the analyses using a timed urine specimen and calculating the free water clearance. The free water clearance is determined by first calculating the osmolar clearance using the standard clearance

formula of $C_{OSM} = \dfrac{U_{OSM} \times V}{P_{OSM}}$ and then subtracting the osmolar clearance value from the

urine volume.

Example: Using (U) urine osmolarity of 600 mOsm, (V) urine volume of 2 ml/min, and (P) plasma osmolarity of 300 mOsm, calculate the free water clearance.

$$C_{OSM} = \frac{600 \, (U) \times 2 \, (V)}{300 \, (P)} = 4.0 \text{ ml/min}$$

$$C_{H_2O} = 2 \, (V) - 4.0 \, (C_{OSM}) = -2.0$$

Calculation of the osmolar clearance tells how much water must be cleared each minute to produce a urine with the same osmolarity as the plasma. Remember that the ultrafiltrate contains the same osmolarity as the plasma; therefore, the osmotic differences found in the urine are the result of renal concentrating and diluting mechanisms. By comparing the osmolar clearance to the actual urine volume excreted per minute, it can be determined if the water being excreted is more or less than the amount needed to maintain an osmolarity the same as the ultrafiltrate. The above calculation shows a free water clearance of −2.0, indicating that less than the necessary amount of water is being excreted and renal concentration is taking place. If the value had been zero, no renal concentration or dilution would be taking place; likewise, if the value had been +2.0, renal dilution would be occurring.[19] Therefore, calculation of the free water clearance can be used to determine the amount and type of work being done by the tubules.

TUBULAR SECRETION AND RENAL BLOOD FLOW TESTS

As discussed earlier, in the tubular secretion process, waste products are removed from the blood in the peritubular capillaries and are transferred into the filtrate by the tubular cells. Without adequate renal blood flow, substances to be secreted will not be properly presented to the tubules; therefore, a test for tubular secretion also becomes a measure of renal blood flow and the number of functional nephrons. To understand the principles and limitations of the tests employed, it then becomes necessary to determine whether impaired tubular secretion or renal blood flow is the cause of the abnormal test result.

PSP TEST

The two tests most commonly associated with tubular secretion and renal blood flow are the phenolsulfonphthalein (PSP) test and the p-aminohippuric acid (PAH) test. Both tests rely on tubular secretion for the measurement of renal blood flow. Phenolsulfonphthalein is a dye. When it is injected into the bloodstream, approximately 94 percent of the dye binds to the plasma proteins. The protein-bound dye cannot be filtered by the glomerulus and must be removed by tubular secretion. PSP dye is secreted in the proximal convoluted tubule, where the dye has a stronger affinity for the cells lining the tubule than it does for the plasma proteins; therefore, it dissociates from the plasma proteins and is secreted into the filtrate by the cells of the proximal convoluted tubule.

The PSP test is performed by injecting 6 mg of phenolsulfonphthalein dye into a well-hydrated patient, collecting urine specimens at 15, 30, 60, and 120 minutes post-injection, and measuring the amount of dye excreted in each specimen. Measurement of the dye concentration is based on the principle that phenolsulfonphthalein produces a pink color in alkaline solutions. The urine specimens are made alkaline with sodium hydroxide and diluted to a uniform volume with distilled water, and the intensity of the pink color is compared to standards of known concentration using a spectrophotometer. Substances that produce a cloudy specimen, such as blood and amorphous crystals, will interfere with the spectrophotometer readings and should be removed by centrifugation prior to performing the test. Patients should also be cautioned to avoid foods that produce highly pigmented urine and to refrain from taking medications for 24 hours prior to the test.[3]

Accurate timing and collection of the specimens are critical because normal values are based on the percentage of dye excreted in the four time periods. The 15-minute specimen is the most informative, since given enough time, even poorly functioning kidneys will excrete the dye. This specimen normally contains about 35 percent of the dye. By the end of the first hour, approximately 60 percent of the dye has been excreted; at the end of 2 hours, 75 percent. Values below 25 percent in the 15-minute specimen indicate impaired renal function. Even though the method of dye removal is tubular secretion and the PSP test is often referred to as a secretion test, the defective function is actually renal blood flow. This is because the small amount of diluted dye presented to the tubules could be secreted even by damaged cells. Therefore, failure to excrete an acceptable amount of the dye in the 15-minute specimen must be attributed to inadequate renal blood flow, which causes a delay in the presentation of the dye to the tubule cells.

PAH TEST

The ease by which the PSP test can be performed has made it a popular screening test for renal blood flow. However, because the dye is not completely removed from the blood during a single pass through the kidney, it cannot be used to determine the actual blood flow in milliliters per minute. To measure the exact amount of blood flowing through the kidney, it is necessary to use a substance that is completely removed from the blood (plasma) each time it comes in contact with functional renal tissue. The principle is the same as in the clearance test for glomerular filtration. However, to ensure measurement of the blood flow through the entire nephron, the substance must be removed from the blood primarily in the peritubular capillaries, rather than being removed when the blood reaches the glomerulus. Although it has the disadvantage of being exogenous, the chemical *p*-aminohippurate meets the criteria needed to measure renal blood flow. It is a nontoxic substance that binds less strongly to plasma proteins than PSP dye, which permits its complete removal as the blood passes through the peritubular capillaries. Approximately 10 percent of the PAH is filtered through the glomerulus; and except for a small amount contained in plasma that does not come in contact with functional renal tissue, the remainder is secreted by the proximal convoluted tubule. As with any clearance test, the amount of PAH excreted in the urine will be determined by the volume of plasma flowing through the kidneys. The standard clearance formula C_{PAH} (ml/min) $= \dfrac{U \text{ (mg/dl PAH)} \times V \text{ (ml/min urine)}}{P \text{ (mg/dl PAH)}}$ can be used to calculate the effective renal plasma flow. Normal values for the effective renal plasma flow range from 600 to 700 ml per min, making the average renal blood flow about 1200 ml per min. Notice that the actual measurement is renal plasma flow rather than renal blood flow, since the PAH is contained only in the plasma portion of the blood. Also, the term "effective" is included because approximately 8 percent of the renal blood flow does not come in contact with the functional renal tissue.[7] The PAH test is not routinely performed in the clinical laboratory due to the difficulty in maintaining a constant infusion level of the exogenous PAH. When necessary, patients with abnormal PSP results are referred to specialized renal laboratories for this procedure. Procedures are currently being developed using radioactively labeled hippurate, which will simplify specimen analysis and can lead to single-injection methods for the measurement of renal blood flow.[22]

TITRATABLE ACIDITY AND URINARY AMMONIA

Both the PSP and PAH tests involve the tubular secretion of foreign substances, but it may also be necessary to evaluate tubular secretion of excess metabolic wastes. Hydrogen ions are the waste product of most concern because the kidney is the major regulator of the acid-base balance in the body. A normal person excretes approximately 70 mEq of acid per day, in the form of either titratable acid (H^+) or ammonium ions (NH^+).[10] Hydrogen ions that are secreted in the proximal and distal convoluted tubules combine either with phosphate and carbonate buffers that are present in the filtrate or with ammonia that is produced and secreted by the tubular cells. Since a patient who is unable to excrete an acidic urine (renal tubular acidosis) may have impaired ammonia production or may lack adequate buffers to transport the hydrogen ions, tests to evaluate titratable acidity and urinary ammonium levels are performed. Tests can be run simultaneously on either fresh or toluene-preserved urine specimens collected at 2-hour intervals from patients who have been primed with an acid load consisting of oral ammonium chloride. By titrating the amount of free H^+ (titratable acidity) and then the total acidity of the specimen, the ammonium concentration can be calculated as the difference between the titratable acidity and the total acidity.[6] In a normal person, approximately two thirds of the excreted acid is ammonium ion and one third is in the form of titratable acid. Variations in the ratio, along with a decrease in total acid excretion, can then be analyzed to determine whether the patient's problem is due to inadequate filtration of buffer, lack of hydrogen secretion, or decreased ammonia production.

RENAL DISEASES

Although disease states throughout the body can affect renal function and produce abnormalities in the urinalysis, abnormal results are frequently associated with disorders directly affecting the kidney. A basic discussion of the major renal diseases including possible causes, clinical symptoms, associated pathology, and laboratory findings (Table 2-2) is presented at this point to enable laboratory personnel to better understand the significance of test results in these conditions.

ACUTE GLOMERULONEPHRITIS

In general, glomerulonephritis refers to a sterile inflammatory process that affects the glomerulus and is associated with the finding of blood, protein, and casts in the urine.[8] Acute glomerulonephritis, as the name implies, is a disease characterized by the rapid onset of symptoms consistent with damage to the glomerular membrane. It is most frequently seen in children and young adults following respiratory tract infections caused by certain strains of group A streptococci. During the course of the infection, these nephrogenic strains of streptococci are believed to form immune complexes with circulating antibodies and become deposited on the glomerular membrane, resulting in damage to the integrity of the membrane. Similar damage can also be produced by exposure to nephrotoxic chemicals.[11] In most cases, successful management of the secondary complications, which include edema, hypertension, and electrolyte imbalance until the inflammation has subsided, will result in a permanent cure. A more serious form of the disease, called crescentic, or rapidly progressive, glomerulonephritis, has a much poorer prognosis, often terminating in renal failure. Crescent formation by epithelial cells on the inside of Bowman's capsule and changes in the glomerular capillary tufts due to fibrin deposition cause breakage of the capillary basement membrane, resulting in permanent damage to the glomeruli.

Primary urinalysis findings include marked hematuria, increased protein, and oliguria, accompanied by red blood cell casts, hyaline and granular casts, and white blood cells. As toxicity to the glomerular membrane subsides, the urinalysis results will return to normal, with the possible exception of microscopic hematuria that lasts until the membrane damage has been repaired. Blood urea nitrogen may be elevated during the acute stages but, like the urinalysis, will return to normal unless the disease develops into rapidly progressive glomerulonephritis. Demonstration of an elevated serum antistreptolysin O titer provides evidence that the disease is of streptococcal origin.

CHRONIC GLOMERULONEPHRITIS

The term chronic glomerulonephritis has been used to describe a variety of disorders that produce continual or permanent damage to the glomerulus. Classifications vary somewhat among authors but primarily include membranous, membranoproliferative, and focal glomerulonephritis, and minimal change disease. Currently, these conditions are categorized separately, and chronic glomerulonephritis is used to represent the end-stage result of persistent glomerular damage associated with irreversible loss of renal tissue and chronic renal failure.[13] Clinical symptoms include edema, hypertension, anemia, metabolic acidosis, and oliguria progressing to anuria. Examination of the urine in chronic glomerulonephritis reveals: the presence of blood, protein, and many varieties of casts, including broad casts; and a specific gravity of 1.010, indicating a loss of renal concentrating ability and a decreased glomerular filtration rate. Blood urea nitrogen and creatinine are elevated, as are the serum phosphorus and potassium. Serum calcium levels are noticeably decreased.

MEMBRANOUS GLOMERULONEPHRITIS

The predominant characteristic of membranous glomerulonephritis is a pronounced thickening of the glomerular capillary basement membrane. In autoimmune diseases, such as systemic lupus erythematosus, deposition of immune complexes on the membrane produces the thickening. However, increased membrane epithelial cell production leading to membrane thickening occurs with secondary syphilis, Sjögren's syndrome, gold and mercury treatments, hepatitis B antigen, and malignancies. Many cases of unknown etiology have also been diagnosed.[11] As a rule, the disease progresses slowly, and remissions are frequent; but the patient may eventually develop a nephrotic syndrome.

Laboratory findings include microscopic hematuria and elevated urine protein excretion that may reach concentrations similar to those in the nephrotic syndrome. Demonstration of systemic lupus erythematosus or hepatitis B through blood tests can aid in the diagnosis.

MEMBRANOPROLIFERATIVE GLOMERULONEPHRITIS

Sometimes referred to as mesangioproliferative glomerulonephritis, this form of glomerulonephritis is characterized by two different alterations in the glomerular cellularity. Type I displays increased cellularity in the subendothelial cells of the mesangium; whereas Type II displays dense deposits thought to be of lipoprotein or immune origin.[1] Many of the patients are children or young adults with previous streptococcal respiratory infections. The clinical course is variable, as are the laboratory findings; however, hematuria, proteinuria, and decreased serum complement levels are frequent findings.

FOCAL GLOMERULONEPHRITIS

In contrast to other forms of glomerulonephritis, focal glomerulonephritis affects only a certain number of glomeruli, while the others remain normal.[12] With the presence of normally functioning nephrons, the clinical course may be less severe than in other forms unless the abnormalities are associated with systemic disorders such as lupus erythematosus and Goodpasture's syndrome. Immune deposits are a frequent finding and are often seen in undamaged glomeruli. Microscopic and macroscopic hematuria and proteinuria are routine laboratory findings.

MINIMAL CHANGE DISEASE

As the name implies, minimal change disease produces little cellular change in the glomerulus. Patients are frequently children who present with edema, heavy proteinuria, lipiduria, and transient hematuria.[1] Although the etiology is unknown at this time, considerable attention is being given to abnormalities in cell-mediated immunity.[8] The prognosis is generally good, with frequent complete remissions.

NEPHROTIC SYNDROME

The nephrotic syndrome is characterized by the appearance of massive proteinuria, edema, high levels of serum lipids, and low levels of serum albumin.[8] Circulatory disorders that affect the pressure and flow of blood to the kidney are one of the most frequent causes of the nephrotic syndrome, and it may occur as a complication in cases of glomerulonephritis. Lipid nephrosis, which is usually seen in children, may be due

TABLE 2-2. Laboratory Correlations in Renal Diseases[11,12,13]

Disease	Routine Urinalysis	Microscopic Examination	Other Laboratory Findings	Remarks
Acute Glomerulonephritis	Macroscopic hematuria Specific gravity ↑ Protein <5 g/day	RBCs RBC casts Granular casts WBCs	ASO titer ↑ GFR ↓ Sedrate ↑	Microscopic hematuria remains longer than proteinuria
Rapidly Progressive (Crescentic) Glomerulonephritis	Macroscopic hematuria Protein	RBCs WBCs Granular casts	BUN ↑ Creatinine ↑ Fibrin degradation products ↑ GFR ↓ Cryoglobulins ↑	Oliguria
Chronic Glomerulonephritis	Macroscopic hematuria Specific gravity 1.010 Protein	RBCs WBCs All types of casts Broad casts	BUN ↑ Creatinine ↑ Serum phosphorus ↑ Serum calcium ↓	Oliguria or anuria Nocturia Anemia
Membranous Glomerulonephritis	Blood Protein	RBCs Hyaline casts	Positive ANA Positive HB_sAg	Microscopic hematuria
Membranoproliferative (Mesangioproliferative) Glomerulonephritis	Macroscopic hematuria Protein	RBCs RBC casts	BUN ↑ Creatinine ↑ ASO titer ↑ Complement ↓	Hematuria may be microscopic
Focal Glomerulonephritis	Blood Protein	RBCs Fat droplets	IgA deposits on membrane	Macroscopic or microscopic hematuria

Minimal Change Disease	Blood	RBCs Oval fat bodies Fat droplets Hyaline casts Fatty casts	Serum protein ↓ Serum albumin ↓	Hematuria may be absent
Nephrotic Syndrome	Protein	Oval fat bodies Fat droplets Generalized casts Waxy casts Fatty casts	Serum lipids ↑ Serum protein ↓ Serum albumin ↓	Heavy proteinuria >5 g/day
Pyelonephritis	Cloudy Protein Nitrite Leukocytes	WBCs WBC casts Bacteria RBCs		Concentrating ability decreased in chronic cases

to an allergic reaction.[24] Tubular damage, as well as glomerular damage, occurs, and the condition may progress to chronic renal failure.

Urinalysis observations include marked proteinuria, urinary fat droplets, oval fat bodies, renal tubular epithelial cells and casts, waxy and fatty casts, or, in general, a telescoped sediment.

RENAL FAILURE

Characterized by failure of the renal excretory mechanism resulting in anuria or oliguria, this is a serious condition. The three major causes of renal failure are renal vasoconstriction, tubular damage, and mechanical obstruction.[23] Hypotension due to traumatic or surgical shock, burns, and acute intravascular hemolysis, as occurs in transfusion reactions, are frequent causes of acute renal failure. Failure due to tubular damage and mechanical obstruction is usually of a more chronic nature, resulting from previous renal disease. Aside from the marked decrease in urine volume, laboratory findings will vary depending on the cause of the failure. In cases involving tubular damage, there will be a lack of concentrating ability and the presence of renal tubular epithelial cells. In contrast, highly concentrated specimens may be found in vascular disorders.[23]

PYELONEPHRITIS

Defined as an infection of the renal tubules, pyelonephritis can exist in both acute and chronic forms. However, pyelonephritis is usually not considered chronic until tubular damage has occurred. Without the presence of tubular damage, even recurrent infections are classified as acute.[24] Pyelonephritis is most frequently seen in women, often resulting from untreated cases of cystitis. Recurrent infections indicate obstruction of the urinary flow, which allows opportunistic bacterial growth because the infected urine remains in the kidney.[17] Congenital structural defects and renal calculi are frequent causes of urinary flow obstruction. Major urinary findings include the presence of white blood cells, often in clumps or casts, bacteria, positive nitrite reactions, and possible proteinuria and hematuria.

REFERENCES

1. ANTONOVYCH, TT: *Atlas of Kidney Biopsies.* Armed Forces Institute of Pathology, Washington, DC, 1980.
2. BARTTER, F AND DELEA, C: *Diabetes insipidus: Its nature and diagnosis.* Laboratory Management 20(1):23–28, 1982.
3. BAUER, JD: *Clinical Laboratory Methods.* CV Mosby, St. Louis, 1982.
4. BIANCHI, C: *Noninvasive methods for the measurement of renal function.* In DUART, C (ED): *Renal Function Tests: Clinical Laboratory Procedures and Diagnosis.* Little, Brown & Co, Boston, 1980.
5. CAMPBELL, J AND CAMPBELL, JB: *Laboratory Mathematics.* CV Mosby, St. Louis, 1980.
6. CHAN, J: *Renal acidosis.* In DUART, C (ED): *Renal Function Tests: Clinical Laboratory Procedures and Diagnosis.* Little, Brown & Co, Boston, 1980.
7. DUSTON, H AND CORCORAN, A: *Functional interpretation of renal tests.* Med Clin North Am 39:947–956, 1955.
8. FORLAND, M (ED): *Nephrology.* Medical Examination Publishing, New York, 1983.
9. FREW, AJ, ET AL: *Estimation of urine specific gravity and osmolality using a simple reagent strip.* Br Med J 285:(6349):1168, 1982.
10. GOODMAN, AD: *New thoughts on renal glyconeogenesis.* In LAULER, D (ED): *Urinalysis in the 70's.* Medcom, New York, 1973.

11. HEPTINSTALL, RH: *Pathology of the Kidney, Vol I.* Little, Brown & Co, Boston, 1983.
12. HEPTINSTALL, RH: *Pathology of the Kidney, Vol II.* Little, Brown & Co, Boston, 1983.
13. HEPTINSTALL, RH: *Pathology of the Kidney, Vol III.* Little, Brown & Co, Boston, 1983.
14. JACOBSEN, FK, ET AL: *Evaluation of kidney function after meals.* Lancet i(8163):319–320, 1980.
15. JAMISON, R AND ROBERTSON, C: *Recent formulations of the urinary concentrating mechanisms: A status report.* Kidney Int 16(5):537–545, 1979.
16. JUEL, R: *Serum osmolality: A CAP survey analysis.* Am J Clin Pathol 68:165–167, 1977.
17. KURTZ, SB: *Urinary tract infection.* In KNOX, FG (ED): *Textbook of Renal Pathophysiology.* JB Lippincott, Philadelphia, 1978.
18. MERCIER, DE, FELD, RD, AND WITTE, DI: *Comparison of dewpoint and freezing point osmometry.* Am J Med Technol 44(11):1066–1069, 1978.
19. MURPHY, JE, PREUSS, HG, AND HENRY, JB: *Evaluation of renal function and water, electrolyte and acid-base balance.* In HENRY, JB (ED): *Clinical Diagnosis and Management by Laboratory Methods.* WB Saunders, Philadelphia, 1984.
20. OKEN, D: *Osmometry and differential diagnosis.* In LAULER, D (ED): *Urinalysis in the 70's.* Medcom, New York, 1973.
21. PRICE, JD AND DURNFORD, J: *Laboratory test for kidney function: Urea or creatinine?* Lancet ii(8140):420–422, 1979.
22. SCHNURR, E, LAHME, W, AND KUPPERS, H: *Measurement of renal clearance of inulin and PAH in the steady state without urine collection.* Clin Nephrol 13(1):26–29, 1980.
23. SIGLER, MH: *Aniguric renal failure and acute tubular necrosis.* Med Clin North Am 47(4):906–926, 1963.
24. *Kidney Diseases: A Guide for Public Health Personnel.* US Department of Health, Education and Welfare, Washington, DC, 1970.
25. WEISBERG, HF: *Osmolality.* Laboratory Medicine 12(2):81–85, 1981.

STUDY QUESTIONS (Choose one best answer)

1. Each kidney is composed of approximately:

   a. 100 nephrons
   b. 1,000 nephrons
   c. 10,000 nephrons
   d. 1,000,000 nephrons

2. The total renal blood flow is approximately:

   a. 60 ml/min
   b. 120 ml/min
   c. 600 ml/min
   d. 1200 ml/min

3. The normal kidney performs all of the following functions except:

   a. removes metabolic waste products from the blood
   b. regulates the acid-base balance in the body
   c. removes excess protein from the blood
   d. regulates the water content in the body

4. The glomerular filtrate is described as:

    a. a protein filtrate of plasma
    b. a glucose- and protein-containing filtrate of plasma
    c. a plasma filtrate without glucose and protein
    d. an ultrafiltrate of plasma that does not contain protein

5. The specific gravity of the fluid leaving the glomerulus is:

    a. 1.001
    b. 1.010
    c. 1.020
    d. 1.030

6. In the proximal convoluted tubule, glucose is reabsorbed by active transport, and urea by passive transport. For active transport to occur:

    a. glucose must combine with a carrier protein, creating electrochemical energy
    b. glucose must be filtered through the tubular membranes
    c. glucose concentration in the tubular filtrate must be higher than in the blood
    d. glucose concentration in the blood must be higher than in the tubular filtrate

7. Active transport of glucose ceases when the renal threshold reaches:

    a. 50–100 mg/dl
    b. 160–180 mg/dl
    c. 220–240 mg/dl
    d. over 240 mg/dl

8. Concentration of the tubular filtrate by the countercurrent mechanism is dependent on all of the following except:

    a. high salt concentration in the renal medulla
    b. water impermeable walls in the ascending loop of Henle
    c. active transport of sodium in the ascending loop of Henle
    d. active transport of glucose and amino acids in the proximal convoluted tubule

9. Aldosterone and ADH are:

    a. hormones that regulate the reabsorption of glucose
    b. hormones that regulate the permeability of the tubular walls in the descending and ascending loops of Henle
    c. hormones that regulate the countercurrent mechanism
    d. hormones that regulate final urine volume and sodium content

10. Substances removed from the blood by tubular secretion include primarily:

    a. protein, hydrogen, and ammonia
    b. protein, hydrogen, and potassium
    c. protein-bound substances, hydrogen, and potassium
    d. amino acids, hydrogen, and ammonia

11. Clearance tests for glomerular filtration must use substances that are:

    a. not filtered by the glomerulus

b. completely reabsorbed in the proximal convoluted tubule

c. secreted in the distal convoluted tubule

d. neither reabsorbed nor secreted by the tubules

12. The creatinine clearance test for glomerular filtration is an:

    a. endogenous procedure
    b. exogenous procedure

13. The most common cause of error in the creatinine clearance test is:

    a. miscalculation of chemical results
    b. variation in serum creatinine levels
    c. improperly collected urine specimens
    d. diet high in vegetables

14. A clearance test is reported as:

    a. milligrams per deciliter
    b. milligrams per 24 hours
    c. milliliters per 24 hours
    d. milliliters per minute

15. Calculate the creatinine clearance of a 6-hour specimen using the following data:

    urine creatinine   = 90 mg/dl
    plasma creatinine = 1.8 mg/dl
    urine volume   = 720 ml

16. A 6-year-old child has a total body surface of 0.86 square meters. Calculate the creatinine clearance from a 4-hour specimen with a volume of 120 ml, urine creatinine of 150 mg/dl, and plasma creatinine of 1.5 mg/dl.

17. John White donates one of his two healthy kidneys to his twin brother. His glomerular filtration rate can be expected to:

    a. decrease by 50 percent
    b. increase by 50 percent
    c. decrease gradually over 1 year
    d. remain essentially unchanged

18. One of the three morning specimens collected in a Fishberg concentration test should have a specific gravity of at least:

    a. 1.002
    b. 1.010
    c. 1.022
    d. 1.034

19. Lack of tubular concentrating ability is indicated when the Mosenthal test shows:

    a. high specific gravity and low volume in the night specimen
    b. low specific gravity and high volume in the night specimen
    c. specific gravity over 1.026 in the day specimen
    d. specific gravity over 1.010 and volume over 300 ml in the night specimen

20. An osmole is defined as:

    a. one gram molecular weight of a substance
    b. one gram equivalent weight of a substance
    c. one gram molecular weight of a substance divided by the number of its disso-
       ciation particles
    d. one gram equivalent weight of a substance divided by the number of its disso-
       ciation particles

21. Measurement of urine osmolarity is a more accurate measure of renal concentrating
    ability than specific gravity measured by urinometer because:

    a. osmolarity is measured by instrumentation
    b. specific gravity is not influenced by urea and glucose molecules
    c. specific gravity measures only urea and glucose concentrations
    d. osmolarity is influenced equally by large and small molecules

22. Osmometers utilizing the freezing point colligative property of solutions are based
    on the principle that:

    a. one osmole of nonionizing substance dissolved in one kilogram of water raises
       the freezing point 1.86°C
    b. one osmole of nonionizing substance dissolved in one kilogram of water lowers
       the freezing point 1.86°C
    c. increased solute concentration will raise the freezing point of water in direct
       proportion to an NaCl standard
    d. decreased solute concentration will decrease the freezing point in direct pro-
       portion to an NaCl standard

23. Vapor pressure osmometers are based on the principle that:

    a. increased solute raises the vapor pressure of a solution
    b. increased solute lowers the dew-point temperature of a solution
    c. increased solute raises the dew-point temperature of a solution
    d. a and c but not b are correct

24. Substances that may interfere with the measurement of urine and serum osmolarity
    include all of the following except:

    a. ethanol
    b. lactic acid
    c. sodium
    d. lipids

25. The normal serum osmolarity is:

    a. 50–100 mOsm
    b. 275–300 mOsm
    c. 400–500 mOsm
    d. 3 times the urine osmolarity

26. A free water clearance of +3.0 could be indicative of:

    a. dehydration
    b. lack of renal concentration and dilution

c. diabetes insipidus

d. increased ADH production

27. The PSP test is used primarily as a measure of:

    a. renal concentration
    b. renal secretion
    c. renal urine flow
    d. glomerular filtration

28. The most informative specimen in the PSP test is the:

    a. 15-minute
    b. 30-minute
    c. 1-hour
    d. 2-hour

29. To provide an accurate measure of renal blood flow, a test substance should be:

    a. completely filtered by the glomerulus
    b. completely reabsorbed by the tubules
    c. completely secreted when it reaches the distal convoluted tubule
    d. completely cleared on each contact with functional renal tissue

30. A steady infusion of *p*-aminohippuric acid is given to a patient over a 1-hour period, and 90 ml of urine are collected during this time. Calculate the patient's renal blood flow using a urine PAH concentration of 360 mg/dl and a plasma PAH concentration of 0.8 mg/dl.

31. Renal tubular acidosis is:

    a. the production of excessively acidic urine due to increased filtration of hydrogen ions
    b. the production of excessively acidic urine due to increased secretion of hydrogen ions
    c. the inability to produce an acidic urine due to impaired production of ammonia
    d. the inability to produce an acidic urine due to the increased production of ammonia

32. Match the following routine urinalysis results with the most probably renal function abnormality:

    _____ 2+ protein   a. decreased ammonia production
    _____ 4+ glucose   b. oliguria
    _____ 1.002 specific gravity   c. proximal convoluted tubule damage
    _____ pH 8.0   d. increased ADH
    _____ broad casts   e. glomerular membrane damage
                                    f. decreased ADH
                                    g. increased renal blood flow

3
PHYSICAL EXAMINATION OF THE URINE

INSTRUCTIONAL OBJECTIVES

Upon completion of this chapter, readers will be able to:

1. list the common terminology used to report normal urine color

2. discuss the relationship of urochrome to normal urine color

3. tell how the presence of bilirubin in a specimen may be suspected

4. discuss the significance of cloudy red urine and clear red urine

5. name two possible causes of black or brown urine

6. discuss the significance of Pyridium in a specimen

7. define appearance

8. list the common terminology used to report appearance

9. describe the appearance and discuss the significance of amorphous phosphates and amorphous urates in freshly voided urine

10. list three pathologic and four nonpathologic causes of cloudy urine

11. define specific gravity and tell why this measurement is valuable in the routine analysis

12. describe the principles of physics used in measuring specific gravity by urinometer and refractometer

13. given the calibration temperature and specimen temperature, calculate a temperature correction for a specific gravity reading determined by urinometer

14. given the concentration of glucose and protein in a specimen, calculate the correction needed to compensate for these high molecular weight substances in the urinometer specific gravity reading

15. name two nonpathogenic causes of abnormally high specific gravity readings

As mentioned in Chapter 1, early physicians based many medical decisions on the color and appearance of urine. Today, observation of these characteristics provides preliminary information concerning disorders such as glomerular bleeding, liver disease, inborn errors of metabolism, and urinary tract infection. Measurement of specific gravity evaluates renal tubular function. The results of the physical portion of the urinalysis can also be used to confirm or explain findings in the chemical and microscopic areas of the urinalysis.

COLOR

The color of urine varies from almost colorless to black. These variations may be due to normal metabolic functions, physical activity, ingested materials, or pathologic conditions. A noticeable change in urine color is often the reason a patient seeks medical advice, and it then becomes the responsibility of the laboratory to determine if this color change is normal or pathologic.

NORMAL URINE COLOR

Terminology used to describe the color of normal urine may differ slightly among laboratories. Common descriptions include pale yellow, straw, light yellow, yellow, dark yellow, and amber. Care should be taken to examine the specimen under a good light source, looking down through the container against a white background. The yellow color of urine is due to the presence of a pigment named urochrome by Thudichum in 1864. Urochrome is a product of endogenous metabolism, and under normal conditions, it is produced at a constant rate. The actual amount of urochrome produced is dependent on the body's metabolic state, with increased amounts being produced in thyroid conditions and fasting states.[3] Urochrome increases in urine that stands at room temperature.[9]

Because urochrome is excreted at a constant rate, the intensity of the yellow color in a fresh urine specimen can give a rough estimate of urine concentration. A dilute urine will be pale yellow, and a concentrated specimen will be dark yellow. Remember that due to variations in the body's state of hydration, these differences in the yellow color of urine are normal.

ABNORMAL URINE COLOR

Dark yellow or amber urine may not always signify a normal concentrated urine but can be caused by the presence of the abnormal pigment bilirubin. If bilirubin is present, it will be detected during the chemical examination; however, its presence is suspected if a yellow foam appears when the specimen is shaken. A urine specimen that contains bilirubin may also contain hepatitis virus. It should be handled with special precautions and disposed of in a container designated for infectious materials.

As can be seen in Table 3-1, abnormal urine colors are as numerous as their causes; however, certain colors are seen more frequently and are of greater clinical significance than others. One of the most common causes of abnormal urine color is the presence of blood. Red is the usual color imparted to urine by blood; but the color may range from pink to black, depending on the amount of blood, the pH of the urine, and the length of contact. Red blood cells remaining in an acidic urine for several hours will produce a brown-black urine due to the denaturation of hemoglobin. A fresh brown-black urine containing red blood cells may also be indicative of glomerular bleeding.[1] Besides red blood cells, two other substances, hemoglobin and myoglobin, produce a red urine and result in a positive chemical test for blood. When red blood cells are present, the urine will be red and cloudy; however, if hemoglobin or myoglobin is present, the specimen is red and clear. It may be possible to distinguish between hemoglobinuria and myoglobinuria by examining the patient's plasma. Hemoglobinuria resulting from the in vivo breakdown of red blood cells is accompanied by red plasma; whereas myoglobin is produced by skeletal muscle and does not affect the color of the plasma. The possibility of hemoglobinuria being produced from the in vitro lysis of red blood cells must also be considered. Chemical tests to distinguish between hemoglobin and myoglobin are available (see Chapter 4). Additional testing is also recommended for urine specimens that turn brown or black upon standing and have negative chemical tests for blood, as they may contain melanin or homogentisic acid (see Chapter 6).

TABLE 3-1. Laboratory Correlation of Urine Color[2]

Color	Cause	Laboratory Correlations
Colorless Straw Pale Yellow	Recent fluid consumption	Commonly observed with random specimens
	Polyuria or diabetes insipidus	Increased 24-hour volume
	Diabetes mellitus	Elevated specific gravity and positive glucose test
Dark Yellow Amber Orange	Concentrated specimen	May be normal after strenuous exercise or in a first morning specimen Dehydration from fever or burns
	Bilirubin	Yellow foam when shaken and positive chemical tests for bile
	Acriflavine	Negative bile tests and possible green fluorescence
	Carrots or vitamin A	Soluble in petroleum ether
	Pyridium	Drug commonly administered for urinary tract infections May have orange foam and thick orange pigment that can obscure or interfere with dipstick readings
	Nitrofurantoin	Antibiotic administered for urinary tract infections
Yellow-Green Yellow-Brown	Bilirubin oxidized to biliverdin	Colored foam in acidic urine, and false-negative chemical tests for bilirubin
	Rhubarb	Seen in acidic urine
Green Blue-Green	*Pseudomonas* infection	Positive urine culture
	Amitriptyline	Antidepressant
	Methocarbamol	Muscle relaxant
	Clorets	None
	Indican	Confirm with Obermayer's test
	Methylene blue	None
Pink Red	Red blood cells	Cloudy urine with positive chemical tests for blood and RBCs visible microscopically
	Hemoglobin	Clear urine with positive chemical tests for blood; plasma may be red
	Myoglobin	Clear urine with positive chemical tests for blood; plasma will be colorless Specific identification tests available
	Porphyrins	Negative chemical tests for blood Detect with Watson-Schwartz screening test or fluorescence under ultraviolet light
	Beets	Alkaline urine of genetically susceptible persons
	Phenolsulfonphthalein	Alkaline urines after PSP test for renal function
	Bromsulphalein	Alkaline urines after BSP test for liver function
	Rhubarb	Seen in alkaline urine

TABLE 3-1. *Continued*

Color	Cause	Laboratory Correlations
	Menstrual contamination	Cloudy specimen with red blood cells, mucus, and clots
	Phenindione	Anticoagulant
Brown Black	Red blood cells oxidized to methemoglobin	Seen in acidic urine after standing; positive chemical test for blood
	Myoglobin	Positive chemical test for blood
	Homogentisic acid (Alkaptonuria)	Seen in alkaline urine after standing; specific tests are available
	Melanin or melanogen	Urine darkens upon standing and reacts with nitroprusside and ferric chloride
	Phenol derivatives	Interferes with copper reduction tests
	Argyrol (antiseptic)	Color disappears with ferric chloride
	Methyldopa or levodopa	Antihypertensive

Many abnormal urine colors are of a nonpathogenic nature and are caused by the ingestion of highly pigmented foods, medications, and vitamins. Eating fresh beets will produce a red urine in certain genetically susceptible persons, and chewing Clorets can result in green urine.[10,4] Also frequently encountered in the urinalysis laboratory is the yellow-orange specimen caused by the administration of Pyridium compounds to persons with urinary tract infections. This thick, orange pigment not only obscures the natural color of the specimen, but also interferes with chemical tests based on color reactions. Recognition of the presence of Pyridium in a specimen is important so that alternate testing procedures can be used.

APPEARANCE

Appearance is a general term that refers to the clarity of a urine specimen. In a routine urinalysis, appearance is determined in the same manner used by the ancient physicians, that is, by visually examining the mixed specimen while holding it in front of a light source. The specimen should, of course, be in a clear container. Since many disposable plastic containers are made of nontransparent plastic, it may be necessary to transfer the specimen. Pouring the specimen into a centrifuge tube and examining it prior to centrifugation can be a time-saving step. Common terminology used to report appearance includes clear, hazy, slightly cloudy, cloudy, turbid, and milky.

NORMAL APPEARANCE

Freshly voided normal urine is usually clear; however, cloudiness due to the precipitation of amorphous phosphates and carbonates may be present in fresh alkaline urine. Amorphous phosphates and carbonates usually appear as white clouds in the specimen. Normal acidic urine may also appear cloudy because of precipitated amorphous urates, calcium oxalate, or uric acid crystals. The cloudiness in acidic urine often resembles brick dust due to the accumulation of the pink pigment, uroerythrin, on the surface of the crystals. Uroerythrin is a normal constituent of urine. The presence of squamous epithelial cells and mucus, particularly in specimens from women, will also result in a hazy but normal urine.

TURBIDITY

Besides amorphous crystals, the four most common substances that cause turbidity in urine are white blood cells, red blood cells, epithelial cells, and bacteria.[12] Other causes

TABLE 3-2. Laboratory Correlations in Urine Turbidity[2]

ACIDIC URINE
Amorphous urates
X-ray contrast media
ALKALINE URINE
Amorphous phosphates, carbonates
SOLUBLE WITH HEAT
Amorphous urates, uric acid crystals
SOLUBLE IN DILUTE ACETIC ACID
Red blood cells
Amorphous phosphates, carbonates
INSOLUBLE IN DILUTE ACETIC ACID
White blood cells
Bacteria, yeast
Spermatozoa
SOLUBLE IN ETHER
Lipids
Lymphatic fluid, chyle

include lipids, sperm, mucus, lymph fluid, crystals, yeast, fecal material, and extraneous contamination, such as talcum powder and X-ray contrast media. Many of these substances are nonpathogenic. However, since white blood cells, red blood cells, and bacteria are indicative of pathogenicity, a fresh, turbid specimen can be a cause for concern. The clarity of a urine specimen certainly provides a key to the microscopic examination results, since the degree of turbidity should correspond with the amount of material observed under the microscope. Questionable causes of urine turbidity can be confirmed by the simple chemical tests shown in Table 3-2.

It must also be kept in mind that a clear urine is not always normal. However, with the increased sensitivity of the routine chemical tests and the current addition of a chemical test for leukocytes, most abnormalities in clear urine will be detected prior to the microscopic analysis. It has even been suggested that by accurately measuring turbidity by means of nephelometry, it may be possible to omit the microscopic examination on routine specimens with no degree of turbidity.[12]

SPECIFIC GRAVITY

The kidney's ability to selectively reabsorb essential chemicals and water from the glomerular filtrate is one of the body's most important functions. The intricate process of reabsorption is often the first renal function to become impaired; therefore, an assessment of the kidney's ability to reabsorb is a necessary component of the routine urinalysis. This evaluation is accomplished by measuring the specific gravity of the specimen. Specific gravity will also detect possible dehydration or abnormalities in antidiuretic hormone and can be used to determine if specimen concentration is adequate to ensure accuracy of chemical tests.[5,6]

Specific gravity is defined as the density of a substance compared with the density of a similar volume of distilled water at a similar temperature. Since urine is actually water that contains dissolved chemicals, the specific gravity of urine is a measure of the density of the dissolved chemicals in the specimen. Therefore, as a measure of specimen density, specific gravity is influenced not only by the number of particles present, but also by their size. Large urea molecules contribute more to the reading than do the small sodium and chloride molecules. Since urea is of less value than sodium and chloride in the evaluation of renal concentrating ability, it may also be necessary to test the specimen's osmolality.[11] This procedure is discussed in Chapter 2. However, for purposes of routine urinalysis, the specific gravity provides valuable preliminary information and can be easily performed using either a urinometer (hydrometer) or a refractometer.

URINOMETER

The urinometer consists of a weighted float attached to a scale that has been calibrated in terms of urine specific gravity (1.000 to 1.040). The weighted float displaces a volume of liquid equal to its weight and has been designed to sink to a level of 1.000 in distilled water. The additional mass provided by the dissolved substances in urine causes the float to displace a smaller volume of urine than distilled water. The level to which the urinometer sinks, as shown in Figure 3-1, is representative of the specimen's mass or specific gravity.

The major disadvantage of using a urinometer to measure specific gravity is that it requires a large volume (10 to 15 ml) of specimen. The container in which the urinometer is floated must be wide enough to allow it to float without touching the sides, and the volume of urine must be sufficient to prevent the urinometer from resting on the bottom. When using the urinometer, an adequate amount of urine is first poured into a proper size container, and the urinometer is then added with a spinning motion. The scale reading is then taken at the bottom of the urine meniscus.

It may also be necessary to correct the urinometer reading for temperature, since urinometers are calibrated to read 1.000 in distilled water at a particular temperature. The calibration temperature is printed on the instrument and is usually about 20°C. If the specimen is cold, 0.001 must be subtracted from the reading for each three degrees that the specimen temperature is below the urinometer calibration temperature. Conversely, 0.001 must be added to the reading for each three degrees that the specimen measures above the calibration temperature.

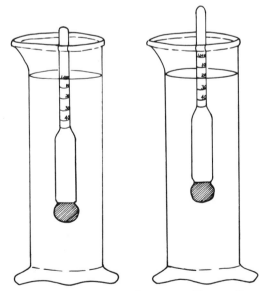

FIGURE 3-1. Urinometers representing various specific gravity readings.

Example: A refrigerated specimen with a temperature of 14°C gives a specific gravity reading of 1.020. Calculate the correct reading.

$$20° \text{ (Calibration Temperature)} - 14° = 6°$$

$$\frac{6°}{3°} \times 0.001 = 0.002$$

$$1.020 - 0.002 = 1.018 \text{ Corrected Specific Gravity}$$

Temperature corrections are not necessary when specific gravity is determined using a refractometer, since readings are automatically temperature corrected.

A correction must also be calculated when using either the urinometer or refractometer if large amounts of glucose or protein are present. Both glucose and protein are high molecular weight substances that have no relationship to renal concentrating ability but will increase specimen density. Therefore, their contribution to the specific gravity is subtracted to give a more accurate report of the kidney's concentrating ability. A gram of protein per deciliter of urine will raise the urine specific gravity by 0.003, and a gram of glucose per deciliter will add 0.004 to the reading. Consequently, for each gram of protein present, 0.003 must be subtracted from the specific gravity reading, and 0.004 must be subtracted for each gram of glucose present.

Example: A. A specimen containing 1 gram of protein and 1 gram of glucose per deciliter has a specific gravity reading of 1.030. Calculate the corrected reading.

$$1.030 - 0.003 \text{ (Protein)} = 1.027 - 0.004 \text{ (Glucose)}$$
$$= 1.023 \text{ Corrected Specific Gravity}$$

B. A refrigerated specimen has a temperature of 17°C and contains 2 grams of protein per deciliter. The urinometer reading is 1.032. Calculate the corrected reading.

$$20° - 17° = 3° = 0.001 \text{ (Temperature Correction)}$$
$$0.003 \times 2 \text{ g} = \underline{0.006} \text{ (Protein Correction)}$$
$$0.007$$

$$1.032 - 0.007 = 1.025 \text{ Corrected Specific Gravity}$$

REFRACTOMETER

The refractometer, like the urinometer, determines the concentration of dissolved particles in a specimen. It does this by measuring refractive index. Refractive index is a comparison of the velocity of light in air with the velocity of light in a solution. The velocity is dependent on the concentration of dissolved particles present in the solution and determines the angle at which light passes through a solution. The clinical refractometer (TS Meter, AO Scientific Instruments Division, Buffalo, New York) makes use of these principles of light by measuring the angle at which light passing through a solution enters a prism and mathematically converting this angle (refractive index) to specific gravity.

The refractometer provides the distinct advantage of determining specific gravity using a small volume of specimen (1 or 2 drops). Temperature corrections are not necessary because the instrument is temperature-compensated between 60°F and 100°F. Corrections for glucose and protein are still calculated, although refractometer readings are less affected by particle density than are urinometer readings.[8] When using the refractometer, a drop of urine is placed on the prism, the instrument is focused at a good light source, and the reading is taken directly from the specific gravity scale (Fig. 3-2). The prism and its cover should be cleaned after each specimen is tested.

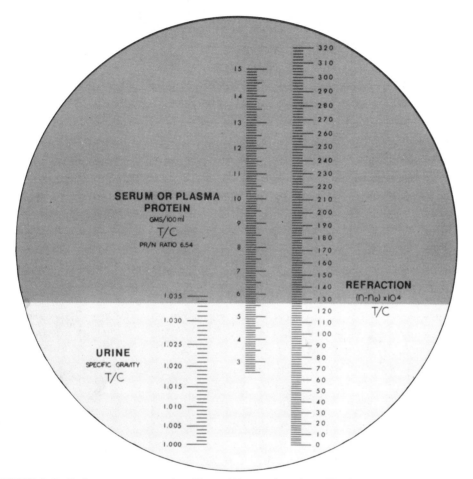

FIGURE 3-2. Refractometer scale. (From Warner Lambert Technologies, Inc., Instructions for Use and Care of the AO TS Meter. Buffalo, New York, with permission. Courtesy of Reichert Scientific Instruments.)

Calibration of the refractometer is performed using distilled water that should read 1.000. If necessary, the instrument contains a zero set screw to adjust the distilled water reading. The calibration is further checked using 5 percent NaCl, which must read 1.022 ± 0.002. Control samples representing low, medium, and high concentrations should also be run at the beginning of each shift. Calibration and control results are always recorded in the appropriate quality control records. A semiautomated instrument (Digital Urinometer, Biovation, Inc., Richmond, California) that employs the principle of refractive index is also available. Specimens are poured across the prism, and readings are displayed on a digital readout screen.

In addition to using the urinometer and refractometer, specific gravity can be determined chemically by dipstick (see Chapter 4) and by the falling drop method. The automated urinalysis instrument (Clinilab, Ames Company, Elkhart, Indiana) uses a falling drop method to measure specific gravity. The instrument determines the amount of time it takes a drop of urine to fall a fixed distance through an insolvent liquid and converts this time to specific gravity.

CLINICAL CORRELATIONS

The specific gravity of the plasma filtrate entering the glomerulus is 1.010. The term isosthenuric is used to describe urine with a specific gravity of 1.010. Specimens below 1.010 are hyposthenuric, and those above 1.010 are hypersthenuric. One would expect urine that has been concentrated by the kidney to be hypersthenuric; however, this is not always true. Normal random specimens may range from 1.001 to 1.035, depending on the patient's degree of hydration. The majority of random specimens fall between 1.015 and 1.025, and any random specimen with a specific gravity of 1.023 or higher is generally considered normal. If a patient exhibits consistently low results, procedures are available for collecting specimens under conditions of controlled fluid intake (see Chapter 2). Abnormally high results, over 1.035, are seen in patients who have recently undergone an intravenous pyelogram. This is caused by the excretion of the injected X-ray contrast media. Patients who are receiving dextran or other high molecular weight intravenous fluids will also produce urine with an abnormally high specific gravity. Once the foreign substance has been cleared from the body, the specific gravity will return to normal. In these circumstances, urine concentration can be measured using the reagent strip chemical test or osmometry.[13] Should the presence of glucose or protein be the cause of high results, this will be detected in the routine chemical examination. As discussed earlier, this can be corrected for mathematically.

ODOR

Although it is seldom of clinical significance and is not a part of the routine urinalysis, urine odor is a noticeable physical property. Freshly voided urine has a faint odor of aromatic compounds. As the specimen stands, the odor of ammonia becomes predominant. The breakdown of urea is responsible for the characteristic ammonia odor. Causes of unusual odors include bacterial infections, which cause a strong, unpleasant odor, and diabetic ketones, which cause a sweet or fruity odor. A serious metabolic defect results in urine with a strong odor of maple syrup and is appropriately called maple syrup urine disease (see Chapter 6). Ingestion of certain foods, particularly asparagus, can cause an unusual or pungent urine odor. Studies have shown that although everyone who eats asparagus produces an odor, only certain genetically predisposed people can smell the odor.[7]

REFERENCES

1. BERMAN, L: *When urine is red.* JAMA 237:2753–2754, 1977.
2. BRADLEY, M AND SCHUMANN, BB: *Examination of the urine.* In HENRY, JB (ED): *Clinical Diagnosis and Management by Laboratory Methods.* WB Saunders, Philadelphia, 1984, p 380 to 458.
3. DRABKIN, DL: *The normal pigment of urine: The relationship of urinary pigment output to diet and metabolism.* J Biol Chem 75:443–479, 1927.
4. EVANS, B: *The greening of urine: Still another "Cloret sign."* N Engl J Med 300(4):202, 1979.
5. FREE, AH: *A Colourimetric method for urine specific gravity compared with current direct and indirect procedures.* Br J Clin Pract 36(9):307–311, 1982.
6. KAVELMAN, DA: *A representative of Ames responds.* Clin Chem 29(1):210–211, 1983.
7. LISON, M, BLONDHEIM, S, AND MELMED, R: *A polymorphism of the ability to smell urinary metabolites of asparagus.* Br Med J 281(6256):1676–1678, 1980.
8. LOW, PS AND TAY, JSH: *Urine: Osmolality refractive index and specific gravity.* J Singapore Paediatr Soc 20(1):37–42, 1978.
9. OSTOW, M AND PHILO, S: *The chief urinary pigment: The relationship between the rate of excretion of the yellow pigment and the metabolic rate.* American Journal of Medical Science 207:507–512, 1944.
10. REIMANN, HA: *Re: Red urine.* JAMA 241(22):2380, 1979.
11. RUBINI, M AND WOLF, AV: *Refractive determination of total solids and water of serum and urine.* J Biol Chem 225:869–876, 1957.

12. SCHUMANN, GB AND GREENBERG, NF: *Usefulness of macroscopic urinalysis as a screening procedure.* Am J Clin Pathol 71(4):452–456, 1979.
13. SMITH, C, ARBOGAST, C, AND PHILLIPS, R: *Effect of X-ray contrast media on results for relative density of urine.* Clin Chem 29(4):730–731, 1983.

STUDY QUESTIONS (Choose one best answer)

1. The normal yellow color of urine is produced by:

   a. bilirubin
   b. urobilinogen
   c. urochrome
   d. hemoglobin

2. A yellow-brown specimen that produces a yellow foam when shaken can be suspected of containing:

   a. bilirubin
   b. hemoglobin
   c. carrots
   d. rhubarb

3. All of the following can contribute to the color of a urine specimen that contains blood except:

   a. amount of blood
   b. type of specimen
   c. pH of specimen
   d. length of contact

4. Specimens that contain intact red blood cells can be visually distinguished from those that contain hemoglobin because:

   a. hemoglobin produces a much brighter red color
   b. hemoglobin produces a cloudy, pink specimen
   c. red blood cells produce a cloudy specimen
   d. red blood cells are quickly converted to hemoglobin

5. After eating beets purchased at the local farmers' market, Mrs. Williams notices that her urine is red, but Mr. Williams's urine remains yellow. The Williamses should:

   a. be concerned because red urine always indicates the presence of blood
   b. not be concerned because all women produce red urine after eating beets
   c. be concerned because they should both have red urine if beets are the cause
   d. not be concerned because only Mrs. Williams is genetically susceptible to producing red urine from beets

6. Specimens from patients receiving treatment for urinary tract infections frequently appear:

   a. clear and red
   b. thick and orange
   c. dilute and pale yellow
   d. cloudy and red

7. Freshly voided urine is normally clear; however, if it is alkaline, a white turbidity may be present due to:

   a. amorphous phosphates and carbonates
   b. white blood cells
   c. uroerythrin
   d. yeast

8. Turbidity in normal acidic urine:

   a. is never observed
   b. is caused by disintegrated epithelial cells
   c. resembles brick dust due to uroerythrin on crystals
   d. resembles a granular white precipitate

9. Which of the following specific gravities would be most likely to correlate with a pale yellow urine?

   a. 1.005
   b. 1.015
   c. 1.025
   d. 1.035

10. Specific gravity is a measure of:

    a. particle content
    b. molecular weight
    c. molarity
    d. density

11. Calculate the corrected specific gravity using the following data:

urinometer reading	= 1.025
urine temperature	= 14°C
urinometer calibration temperature	= 20°C
urine glucose	= 2.0 g/dl
urine protein	= 2000 mg/dl

12. A urine specific gravity measured by refractometer is 1.029, and the temperature of the urine is 14°C. The specific gravity should be reported as:

    a. 1.019
    b. 1.026
    c. 1.029
    d. 1.032

13. Refractive index compares:

    a. light velocity in solutions with light velocity in solids
    b. light velocity in air with light velocity in solutions
    c. light scattering by air with light scattering by solutions
    d. light scattering by particles in solution

14. Refractometers are calibrated using:

    a. distilled water and protein
    b. distilled water and glucose
    c. distilled water and sodium chloride
    d. distilled water and urea

15. A correlation exists between a specific gravity of 1.050 and a:

    a. 2+ glucose
    b. 2+ protein
    c. first morning specimen
    d. radiographic dye infusion

16. An alkaline urine turns black upon standing, develops a cloudy white precipitate, and has a specific gravity of 1.022. The major concern about this specimen would be:

    a. color
    b. turbidity
    c. specific gravity
    d. all of the above

4
CHEMICAL EXAMINATION OF THE URINE

INSTRUCTIONAL OBJECTIVES

Upon completion of this chapter, readers will be able to:

1. describe the proper technique for performing chemical tests on urine by dipstick and give possible errors if this technique is not followed

2. list four causes of premature deterioration of dipsticks and tell how to avoid them

3. list five quality control procedures routinely performed with dipstick testing

4. name two reasons for measuring urinary pH and discuss their clinical applications

5. discuss the principle of pH testing by dipstick

6. describe three renal causes of proteinuria and two nonrenal reasons for proteinuria

7. explain the "protein error of indicators" and list any sources of interference that may occur with this method of protein testing

8. name two confirmatory tests for urine protein performed in the urinalysis laboratory and name any sources of error associated with these procedures

9. describe the unique solubility characteristics of Bence Jones protein and tell how they can be used to perform a screening test for the presence of this protein

10. explain why glucose that is normally reabsorbed in the proximal convoluted tubule may appear in the urine

11. state the renal threshold levels for glucose

12. describe the principle of the glucose oxidase method of dipstick testing for glucose and name possible causes of interference with this method

13. describe the copper reduction method for urinary carbohydrate testing and list possible causes of interference

14. contrast the advantages and disadvantages of the glucose oxidase and copper reduction methods of glucose testing

15. name three reasons for the appearance of ketonuria

16. list the three "ketone bodies" appearing in urine and describe their measurement by the sodium nitroprusside reaction and possible causes of interference

17. differentiate between hematuria and hemoglobinuria and explain the clinical significance

18. describe the chemical principle of the dipstick method for blood testing and list possible causes of interference

19. discuss the presence of myoglobin and its role in the chemical testing for urinary blood

20. describe the degradation of hemoglobin to bilirubin, urobilinogen, and finally urobilin

21. differentiate between conjugated and unconjugated bilirubin, including their relationship to urinary excretion of bilirubin

22. describe the relationship of urinary bilirubin and urobilinogen to the diagnosis of bile duct obstruction, liver disease, and hemolytic disorders

23. name the earliest test to detect urinary bilirubin

24. discuss the principle of oxidation tests and diazotization tests for urinary bilirubin, including possible sources of error

25. tell the advantage of performing an Ictotest for detection of urine bilirubin

26. name two technical errors that may produce false-negative bilirubin reactions

27. give two reasons for increased urine urobilinogen and one reason for an absence of urine urobilinogen

28. name the chemical contained in Ehrlich's reagent

29. give the proper method for collecting and preserving specimens to be tested for urine urobilinogen

30. describe the Watson-Schwartz test used to differentiate among urobilinogen, porphobilinogen, and Ehrlich-reactive compounds

31. Discuss the principle of the nitrite dipstick test for bacteriuria

32. list three possible causes of a false-negative result in the dipstick test for nitrite

33. compare dipstick testing for urine specific gravity with urinometer and refractometer testing

34. give the principle of the chemical dipstick test for leukocytes

35. discuss the advantages and disadvantages of the dipstick test for leukocytes

DIPSTICKS

Routine chemical examination of the urine has changed dramatically since the early days of urine testing due to the development of the dipstick method for chemical analysis. Dipsticks currently provide a simple, rapid means for performing 10 medically significant chemical analyses, including pH, protein, glucose, ketones, blood, bilirubin, urobilinogen, nitrite, specific gravity, and leukocytes (Table 4-1). The two major types of dipsticks are manufactured under the tradenames "Multistix" (Ames Company, Elkhart, Indiana) and "Chemstrip" (Bio-Dynamics/BMC, Indianapolis, Indiana) (Table 4-2). These products are available with single- or multiple-testing areas, and the brand and

TABLE 4-1. Summary of Chemical Testing by Dipsticks

Test	Principle	Interfering Substances	Correlations With Other Tests
pH	Double-indicator system	None	Microscopic Nitrite
Protein	Protein error of indicators	Quaternary ammonium compounds, detergents, and increased salt	Blood Leukocytes Nitrite Microscopic
Glucose	Glucose oxidase, double sequential enzyme reaction	Peroxide, oxidizing detergents, ascorbic acid, 5-HIAA, homogentisic acid, aspirin, and levodopa	Ketones
Ketones	Sodium nitroprusside reaction	Levodopa, phthalein dyes, phenylketones, and 8-hydroxyquinoline	Glucose
Blood	Pseudoperoxidase activity of hemoglobin	Ascorbic acid, nitrite, protein, myoglobin, and oxidizing detergents	Protein Microscopic
Bilirubin	Diazo reaction	Ascorbic acid and nitrite	Urobilinogen
Urobilinogen	Ehrlich's reaction	Porphobilinogen, indican, p-aminosalicylic acid, and sulfonamides	Bilirubin
Nitrite	Griess's reaction	Ascorbic acid	Protein Leukocytes Microscopic
Specific Gravity	pK Change of polyelectrolyte	Glucose, urea, and protein	None
Leukocytes	Granulocytic esterases reaction	Strong oxidizing detergents, ascorbic acid, and proteins	Nitrite Protein Microscopic

number of tests used are a matter of laboratory preference. Dipsticks consist of chemical-impregnated absorbent pads attached to a plastic strip. A color-producing chemical reaction takes place when the absorbent pad comes in contact with urine. Color reactions are interpreted by comparing the color produced on the pad with a chart supplied by the manufacturer. Several colors or intensities of a color for each substance being tested appear on the chart. By careful comparison of the colors on the chart and the stick, a semi-quantitative value of trace, 1+, 2+, 3+, or 4+ can be reported. An estimate of the milligrams per deciliter present is also available for appropriate testing areas on both products.

DIPSTICK TECHNIQUE

Testing methodology consists of: dipping the stick completely, but briefly, into a well-mixed urine specimen; removing excess urine by touching the edge of the strip to the container as the strip is withdrawn; waiting the specified amount of time for the reaction to occur; and comparing the strip to the color chart. Even though this is a simple procedure, improper technique can result in errors. Allowing the stick to remain in the urine for an extended period of time may cause leaching of reagents from the pads. Likewise, excess urine remaining on the stick after its removal from the specimen can produce a run-over between chemicals on adjacent pads, which can result in distortion of the colors. To ensure against run-over, inert absorbent pads have been placed between the affected areas. Holding the strip horizontally while comparing it with the color chart is recommended. The amount of time needed for reactions to take place varies between tests and manufacturers and ranges from an immediate reaction to 60 seconds later. For the best semi-quantitative results, the manufacturer's stated time should be followed; however, when precise timing cannot be adhered to, it is recommended that reactions be read at 60 seconds but never later than 120 seconds.[3] A good light source is, of course, essential for accurate interpretations of color reactions.

QUALITY CONTROL AND STORAGE OF DIPSTICKS

In addition to the use of correct testing technique, dipsticks must be protected from deterioration caused by moisture, volatile chemicals, heat, and light. Both brands of dipsticks are packaged in opaque containers with desiccant, and when not in use, these bottles should be stored tightly closed in a cool area. Bottles should not be opened in the presence of volatile fumes. All bottles are stamped with an expiration date that represents the functional life expectancy of the chemical pads. This date must be honored even if there is no noticeable deterioration of the reagents. Bottles that have been opened for 6 months should also be discarded regardless of the expiration date. Unexpired sticks that have been open for less than 6 months should be visually examined for discoloration and tested for chemical reactivity with controls of known normal and abnormal concentrations. Several commercial controls are available for evaluating dipstick reactivity, and many methods for preparing and preserving urine specimens of known concentrations have been published.[15] Quality control is as important in urinalysis as it is in other sections of the laboratory and must not be neglected. Personnel from each laboratory shift should test dipsticks from open bottles with both positive and negative controls, compare the values, and record them. A check should also be made whenever a new bottle of dipsticks is opened. Results that do not agree with the published control values must be resolved through the testing of additional dipsticks and controls. Demonstration of chemically acceptable dipsticks does not entirely rule out the possibility of inaccurate results. Interfering substances in the urine, technical carelessness, and color blindness will also produce errors. Both dipstick manufacturers have published information concerning the limitations of their chemical reactions, and personnel should be aware of these conditions. As mentioned in Chapter 3, a primary example of dipstick interference is the masking of color reactions by the orange pigment

TABLE 4-2. Comparison of Reagents and Sensitivity of Multistix and Chemstrip[30,38]

Test	Multistix		Chemstrip	
	Reagents	*Sensitivity*	*Reagents*	*Sensitivity*
pH	Methyl red Bromthymol blue	pH 5–9	Methyl red Bromthymol blue Phenolphthalein	pH 5–9
Protein	Tetrabromphenol blue	5–20 mg/dl	3′,3″,5′,5″- Tetrachlorophenol-3,4,5,6- tetrabromosulfophthalein	6 mg/dl
Glucose	Glucose oxidase Peroxidase	100 mg/dl	Glucose oxidase Peroxidase 3-Amino-6-chloro-9- dimethyl-aminopropyl- carbazol-dihydrochloride	40 mg/dl
Ketone	Sodium nitroprusside	5–10 mg/dl Acetoacetic acid	Sodium nitroprusside Glycine	9 mg/dl Acetoacetic acid 40 mg/dl Acetone

Test	Reagents	Range	Reagents (alt.)	Sensitivity
Bilirubin	2, 4 Dichloroaniline diazonium salt	0.2–0.4 mg/dl	2,6-Dichlorobenzene-diazonium-tetrafluoroborate	0.5 mg/dl
Blood	Cumene hydroperoxide Tetramethylbenzidine	0.015–0.062 mg/dl Free hemoglobin 5–20 RBCs	Tetramethylbenzidine 2,5-Dimethyl-2,5-dihydroperoxyhexane	5 RBC/μl Hemoglobin from 10 RBC/μl
Urobilinogen	Para-dimethylaminobenzaldehyde	0.1–1.0 Ehrlich Units	4-Methoxybenzene-diazonium-tetrafluoroborate	0.4 mg/dl
Nitrite	Para-arsanilic acid 1,2,3,4-Tetrahydrobenzo(h)-quinolin-3-01	40–80%	3-Hydroxy-1,2,3,4-tetrahydro-7,8-benzoquinoline Sulfanilamide	1% False
Leukocytes			Indoxycarbonic acid ester Diazonium salt	97.2% Sensitivity
Specific Gravity	Poly(methylvinyl ether maleic anhydride) Bromthymol blue	1.000–1.030		

present in the urine of persons taking Pyridium compounds. If laboratory personnel do not recognize the presence of this pigment, many erroneous results will be reported. Additional or confirmatory procedures employing different chemical principles must be available for the substances being tested by dipstick and should be used when questionable results are obtained or, in some instances, to confirm all positive results. As with dipsticks, the chemical reliability of these procedures must also be checked using positive and negative controls. Specific confirmatory tests and interfering substances are discussed in this chapter under the sections devoted to individual tests.

SUMMARY OF URINARY DIPSTICKS

CARE OF DIPSTICKS

1. Store with desiccant in an opaque, tightly closed container.
2. Store in a cool place, but do not refrigerate.
3. Do not expose to volatile fumes.
4. Do not use past the expiration date.
5. Use within 6 months after opening.
6. Do not use if chemical pads become discolored.

TECHNIQUE

1. Mix specimen well.
2. Dip completely, but briefly, into specimen.
3. Remove excess urine when withdrawing stick from specimen.
4. Compare reaction colors with manufacturer's chart under a good light source at the specified time.
5. Perform confirmatory tests when indicated.
6. Be alert for the presence of interfering substances.
7. Understand the principles and significance of the tests.
8. Relate chemical findings to each other and to the physical and microscopic urinalysis results.

QUALITY CONTROL

1. Test open bottles of dipsticks with known positive and negative controls during each laboratory shift.
2. Resolve control results that are out of range by further testing.
3. Test reagents used in confirmatory tests with positive and negative controls.
4. Perform positive and negative controls on new reagents and dipsticks.
5. Record all control results and reagent lot numbers.

AUTOMATION IN URINALYSIS

Many studies have been done to determine if one brand of dipstick produces fewer errors than the other, and the results have been inconclusive with respect to the quality of the dipsticks. Table 4-2 provides a comparison of the reagents and the sensitivity of the two brands of dipsticks. These same studies have shown that the biggest variable is the conscientiousness of the laboratory personnel in their interpretations of the color reactions.[16] This subjectivity associated with visual discrimination among colors has been alleviated by the development of a semiautomated instrument for the reading of dipsticks. Clini-Tek (Ames Company, Elkhart, Indiana) measures light reflected from a reagent strip that has been manually dipped in urine and inserted into the machine. Light reflection from the test pads decreases in proportion to the intensity of color produced by the concentration of the test substance.[29] Therefore, the instrument compares the amount of light reflection to that of known concentrations and displays or prints concentration units. An automated instrument for reading dipsticks and performing specific gravity utilizes the principle of light reflection for chemical reactions and the falling drop method for specific gravity measurement. The Clinilab (Ames Company, Elkhart, Indiana) adds urine, from vials placed in the machine, to the dipsticks, performs the test for specific gravity, and provides printed results. Instrumentation does not improve the chemical methodology of dipsticks, only the reproducibility and color discrimination.[28] Quality control of the reagent strips must also be performed on a regular basis when using automated systems.

pH

Along with the lungs, the kidneys are the major regulators of the acid-base content in the body. They do this through the secretion of hydrogen in the form of ammonium ion, hydrogen phosphate, and weak organic acids, and by the reabsorption of bicarbonate from the filtrate in the convoluted tubules. Although a healthy individual will usually produce a first morning specimen with a slightly acidic pH of 5.0 to 6.0, the pH of normal random samples can range from 4.5 to 8.0. Consequently, there are no normal values assigned to urinary pH, and it must be considered in conjunction with other patient information, such as the acid-base content of the blood, the patient's renal function, the presence of a urinary tract infection, the patient's dietary intake, and the specimen's age.

CLINICAL SIGNIFICANCE

The importance of urinary pH lies primarily as an aid in determining the existence of systemic acid-base disorders of metabolic or respiratory origin and in the management of urinary conditions that require the urine to be maintained at a specific pH. In respiratory or metabolic acidosis not related to renal function disorders, an acidic urine will be produced; conversely, if respiratory or metabolic alkalosis is present, the urine will be alkaline. Therefore, a urinary pH that does not conform to this pattern may be used to rule out the suspected condition or, as discussed in Chapter 2, may indicate a disorder resulting from the kidneys' inability to secrete or reabsorb acid or base. Urinary crystals and renal calculi are formed by the precipitation of inorganic chemicals dissolved in the urine. This precipitation is dependent on urinary pH and can be controlled by maintaining the urine at a pH that is incompatible with the precipitation of the particular chemicals causing the calculi formation. Knowledge of urinary pH is important in the identification of crystals observed during microscopic examination of the urine sediment. This will be discussed in detail in Chapter 5. The maintenance of an acidic urine can be of value in the treatment of urinary tract infections caused by urea-splitting organisms because they do not multiply as readily in an acidic medium. These same organisms are also responsible for the highly alkaline pH found in specimens that have been allowed to sit unpreserved for extended periods of time. Urinary pH is controlled primarily by dietary regulation, although medications also may be used. Persons on high protein and meat diets tend to produce acidic urine; whereas urine from vegetarians is more alkaline due to the formation of bicarbonate by many fruits and vegetables.[32] An exception to this rule is cranberry juice, which produces an acidic urine and has long been used as a home remedy for minor bladder infections.[20]

SUMMARY OF CLINICAL SIGNIFICANCE OF URINE pH
1. Respiratory or metabolic acidosis causes acidic urine
2. Respiratory or metabolic alkalosis causes alkaline urine
3. Defects in renal tubular secretion and reabsorption of acids and bases
4. Precipitation of crystals and calculi formation
5. Treatment of urinary tract infections
6. Determination of unsatisfactory specimens

DIPSTICK REACTIONS

Both the Multistix and Chemstrip brands of dipstick measure urine pH in 1-unit increments between pH 5 and 9. Because the pH of freshly excreted urine does not reach a pH of 9 in normal or abnormal conditions, a pH of 9 is associated with an improperly preserved specimen and indicates that a fresh specimen should be obtained to ensure the validity of the analysis. To provide differentiation of pH units throughout this wide range, a double-indicator system that consists of methyl red and bromthymol blue is used by both manufacturers. Methyl red is active in the pH range 4.4 to 6.2, producing a color change from red to yellow; bromthymol blue turns from yellow to blue in the pH range 6.0 to 7.6.[21] Therefore, in the pH range 5 to 9 measured by the dipsticks, one will see colors progressing from orange at pH 5 through yellow and green to a final deep blue at pH 9. No known substances interfere with urinary pH measurements performed by dipsticks. However, care must be taken to prevent run-over between the pH testing area and the adjacent, highly acidic protein testing area, as this may produce a falsely acidic reading in an alkaline urine.

PROTEIN

Of the routine chemical tests performed on urine, the most indicative of renal disease is the protein determination. The presence of proteinuria is often associated with early renal disease, making the urinary protein test an important part of any physical examination. Normal urine contains very little protein; usually, less than 150 mg are excreted per 24 hours. This protein consists primarily of low molecular weight serum proteins that have been selectively filtered by the glomerulus and proteins produced in the genitourinary tract. Due to its low molecular weight, albumin is the major serum protein found in normal urine. However, even though it is present in high concentrations in the plasma, the normal urinary albumin content is low because not all of the albumin presented to the glomerulus is actually filtered, and much of the filtered albumin is reabsorbed by the tubules. Other proteins include small amounts of serum and tubular microglobulins, Tamm-Horsfall protein produced by the tubules, and proteins from prostatic, seminal, and vaginal secretions.

CLINICAL SIGNIFICANCE

Demonstration of proteinuria in a routine analysis does not always signify renal disease; however, its presence does require additional testing to determine if the protein represents a normal or a pathologic condition. Major pathologic causes of proteinuria include glomerular membrane damage, disorders affecting tubular reabsorption of filtered protein, and increased serum levels of low molecular weight proteins. When the glomerular membrane is damaged, selective filtration is impaired, and increased amounts of serum albumin and large serum globulin molecules pass through the membrane and are excreted in the urine. Conditions that present the glomerular membrane with abnormal substances (e.g., the immune complexes found in lupus erythematosus and streptococcal glomerulonephritis, amyloid material and toxic agents) are the major causes of proteinuria due to glomerular damage. Increased albumin is also present in disorders that affect tubular reabsorption; however, in contrast to glomerular membrane damage, it is accompanied by other low molecular weight proteins of both serum and tubular origin.[19] The amount of protein that appears in the urine following glomerular damage will range from slightly above normal to 40 grams per day; whereas markedly elevated protein levels are seldom seen in tubular disorders.[31] A primary example of proteinuria due to increased serum protein levels is the excretion of Bence Jones protein by persons with multiple myeloma. In multiple myeloma, a proliferative disorder of the immunoglobulin-producing plasma cells, the serum contains markedly elevated levels of monoclonal immunoglobulin light chains (Bence Jones protein). The low molecular weight protein is filtered in quantities exceeding the tubular reabsorption capacity and is excreted in the urine. Bence Jones protein is a unique protein because, unlike other proteins, it is soluble in urine heated to 100°C. Utilization of this property for chemical testing is discussed later in this section. Identification and quantitation of other urinary proteins are performed using electrophoresis and immunologic techniques. These same techniques should also be used as confirmatory procedures in the analysis of Bence Jones protein.

ORTHOSTATIC (POSTURAL) PROTEINURIA

The discovery of protein, particularly in a random sample, is not always of pathologic significance since several nonpathologic or benign causes of proteinuria exist. Benign proteinuria is usually transient and can be produced by conditions such as exposure to cold, strenuous exercise, high fever, and dehydration. It will disappear when the underlying cause is removed. A more persistent benign proteinuria occurs frequently in young adults and is termed orthostatic, or postural, proteinuria. In these persons, the appearance of urinary protein is related to body position, with proteinuria occurring following periods spent in a vertical posture and disappearing when a horizontal position is assumed. Increased pressure on the renal vein when in the vertical position is believed to account for this condition.[17] Patients suspected of orthostatic proteinuria are requested to collect a specimen immediately upon arising in the morning and a second specimen after remaining in a vertical position for several hours. Both specimens are tested for protein, and if orthostatic proteinuria is present, a negative reading will be seen on the first morning specimen and a positive result will be found on the second specimen. Transient proteinuria not related to renal disease is also often observed during the acute phase of severe illnesses. Proteinuria that occurs during the latter months of pregnancy may indicate a preeclamptic state and should be considered in conjunction with other clinical symptoms to determine if such a problem exists.

DIPSTICK REACTIONS

Dipstick testing for protein utilizes the principle of the "protein error of indicators" to produce a visible colorimetric reaction. Contrary to the general belief that indicators produce specific colors in response to particular pH levels, certain indicators change color in the presence or absence of protein even though the pH of the medium remains constant. Depending on the manufacturer, the protein area of the dipstick contains either tetrabromphenol blue or 3',3",5',5"-tetrachlorophenol-3,4,5,6-tetrabromosulfon-phthalein and an acid buffer to maintain the pH at a constant level. At a pH level of 3, both indicators will appear yellow in the absence of protein; however, as the protein concentration increases, the color will progress through various shades of green and finally to blue. Readings are usually reported in terms of negative, trace, 1+, 2+, 3+, and 4+; however, a semiquantitative value in milligrams per deciliter corresponding to each color change is also supplied by the manufacturers. The protein area of the dipsticks is one of the most difficult to interpret, particularly in relation to the "trace" reading. For this reason, along with the fact that dipsticks primarily measure albumin and may not detect tubular proteins and Bence Jones protein, most laboratories confirm all positive or questionable protein results with the heat or acid precipitation methods. An immunologic method that detects albumin at lower quantities than dipsticks has recently been developed and is being used for monitoring diabetic patients.[39] A positive test for protein will often be found in conjunction with a positive reaction in the blood portion of the dipstick and the finding of casts, red blood cells, white blood cells, or bacteria in the microscopic examination. However, it is possible to have a negative protein in the presence of a small number of casts or blood cells.

PRECIPITATION TESTS

The earliest precipitation tests used heat to denature the protein and produce precipitation; however, other nonprotein substances found in urine are also precipitated by heat. Therefore, acetic acid is added to the heated tube to clear the interfering substances, and sodium chloride is added to ensure protein precipitation in dilute specimens. Currently, most laboratories have replaced the heat and acid test with the less cumbersome cold protein precipitation using sulfosalicylic acid. Various concentrations and amounts of sulfosalicylic acid can be used to precipitate protein, and methods vary greatly among laboratories. By setting up standard curves using known protein concentrations, this method can be adapted to a quantitative procedure, and the amount of precipitation produced can be measured visually against a set of standards or by spectrophotometry or nephelometry. Using this method and a 24-hour urine specimen, the daily output of protein can be determined.

INTERFERING SUBSTANCES

Substances and conditions that produce interference in either the dipstick or the precipitation method are minimal. The major source of error with dipsticks occurs with highly alkaline urine that overrides the buffer system, producing a rise in pH and a color change unrelated to protein concentration. Likewise, a technical error of allowing the reagent pad to remain in contact with the urine for a prolonged period of time may remove the buffer, producing a false-positive reaction. Contamination of the specimen container with quaternary ammonium compounds and detergents may also cause false-positive reactions. High salt concentrations lower the sensitivity of the dipstick.[12] Any substance precipitated by heat and acid will, of course, produce false turbidity in the sulfosalicylic acid test. The most frequently encountered substances are radiographic dyes and tolbutamide metabolites. The presence of radiographic material can be suspected when a markedly elevated specific gravity is obtained and the precipitate increases on standing but dissolves in acetic acid. The patient's history will provide the necessary information on tolbutamide ingestion. As in the dipstick test, a highly alkaline urine may alter the desired acidic pH; however, in this instance, a false-negative reaction will occur because the higher pH will not produce optimum precipitation. All precipitation tests should be performed on centrifuged specimens to remove any extraneous turbidity.

BENCE JONES PROTEIN

When Bence Jones protein is suspected, a screening test that utilizes the unique solubility characteristics of the protein can be performed. Unlike other proteins, which coagulate and remain coagulated when exposed to heat, Bence Jones protein coagulates at temperatures between 40°C and 60°C and dissolves when the temperature reaches 100°C. Therefore, a specimen that appears turbid between 40°C and 60°C and clear at 100°C can be suspected of containing Bence Jones protein. Interference due to other precipitated proteins can be removed by filtering the specimen at 100°C and observing the specimen for turbidity as it cools to between 40°C and 60°C. Not all persons with multiple myeloma produce detectable Bence Jones protein in the urine, and as mentioned earlier, all suspected cases should have protein and immunoelectrophoresis performed on both serum and urine.

SUMMARY OF CLINICAL SIGNIFICANCE OF URINE PROTEIN

1. Glomerular membrane damage
   Immune complex disorders
   Amyloidosis
   Toxic agents
2. Impaired tubular reabsorption
3. Multiple myeloma
4. Orthostatic or postural proteinuria
5. Preeclampsia
6. Diabetic neuropathy

GLUCOSE

Due to its value in the detection and monitoring of diabetes melitus, the glucose test is the most frequent chemical analysis performed on urine. It is estimated that due to the nonspecific symptoms associated with the onset of diabetes, over half of the cases in the world are undiagnosed.[38] Therefore, urine glucose tests are included in all physical examinations and are often the focus of mass health screening programs. Early diagnosis through blood and urine glucose tests provides a greatly improved prognosis. Using currently available dipstick and tablet testing methods, patients can monitor themselves at home and can detect regulatory problems prior to the development of serious complications. It is also recommended that these patients monitor their urinary protein excretion for early detection of diabetic neuropathy.[27]

CLINICAL SIGNIFICANCE

Under normal circumstances, almost all of the glucose filtered by the glomerulus is reabsorbed in the proximal convoluted tubule; therefore, urine contains only minute amounts of glucose. Tubular reabsorption of glucose is by active transport in response to the body's need to maintain an adequate concentration of glucose. Should the blood level of glucose become elevated, as occurs in diabetes mellitus, the tubular transport of glucose ceases and glucose appears in the urine. The blood level at which tubular reabsorption stops is termed the "renal threshold," which for glucose is between 160 and 180 mg per dl. Keep in mind that blood glucose levels will fluctuate, and a normal person may have glycosuria following a meal with a high glucose content. Therefore, the most informative glucose results are obtained from specimens collected under controlled conditions. Fasting prior to the collection of samples for screening tests is recommended. For purposes of diabetes monitoring, specimens are usually tested 2 hours after meals. A first morning specimen does not always represent a fasting specimen because glucose from an evening meal may remain in the bladder overnight, and patients should be advised to empty the bladder and collect the second specimen.[11] Urine for glucose testing is also collected in conjunction with the blood samples drawn during the course of a glucose tolerance test, which is used to confirm the diagnosis of diabetes mellitus. Glycosuria that is not accompanied by elevated blood glucose levels will be seen in conditions that affect tubular reabsorption. It is also found in instances of nondiabetic hyperglycemia, such as occur with central nervous system damage and thyroid disorders. Many pregnant women who may be latent diabetics develop glycosuria during the third trimester and require careful monitoring to determine if it is actually diabetes.

SUMMARY OF CLINICAL SIGNIFICANCE OF URINE GLUCOSE

1. Diabetes mellitus
2. Impaired tubular reabsorption
    Fanconi's syndrome
    Advanced renal disease
3. Central nervous system damage
4. Pregnancy with possible latent diabetes mellitus

GLUCOSE OXIDASE TEST

Two very different tests are utilized by laboratories to measure urinary glucose. The glucose oxidase procedure provides a specific test for glucose, and the copper reduction test is a general test for glucose and other reducing substances. Dipsticks employ the glucose oxidase testing method by impregnating the testing area with a mixture of glucose oxidase, peroxidase, chromogen, and buffer to produce a double sequential enzyme reaction. In the first step, glucose oxidase catalyzes a reaction between glucose and room air to produce gluconic acid and peroxide. Secondly, peroxidase catalyzes the reaction between peroxide and chromogen to form an oxidized colored compound that represents the presence of glucose.

1. $Glucose + O_2 \; (air) \xrightarrow[\text{oxidase}]{\text{glucose}} Gluconic \; Acid + H_2O_2$

2. $H_2O_2 + Chromogen \xrightarrow{\text{peroxidase}} Oxidized \; Colored \; Chromogen + H_2O$

Several different chromogens are used by the dipstick manufacturers, including: o-tolidine, potassium iodide complexes, and 3-amino-6-chloro-9-dimethyl-aminopropyl-carbazol-dihydrochloride. The latter two chromogens provide more distinct differentiation of colors, thereby offering a better means to semiquantitate results. Most laboratories report urine glucose in terms of trace, 1+, 2+, 3+, and 4+; however, the color charts also provide quantitative measurements ranging from 100 mg per dl to 2 g per dl, or 0.1 percent to 2 percent, as recommended by the American Diabetic Association. The sensitivity of the dipsticks has been established at approximately 50 to 100 mg per dl so as not to detect the small amount of glucose normally found in urine.

INTERFERING SUBSTANCES

Because the glucose oxidase method is specific for glucose, false-positive reactions will not be obtained from other urinary constituents, including other sugars that may be present. However, false-positive reactions may occur if containers become contaminated with peroxide or strong oxidizing detergents. Likewise, substances that interfere with the enzymatic reaction or reducing agents that prevent oxidation of the chromogen will produce false-negative results. These include ascorbic acid, 5-hydroxyindoleacetic acid, homogentisic acid, aspirin, and levodopa.[6] High levels of ketones also affect glucose oxidase tests at low glucose concentrations; however, since ketones are usually accompanied by marked glycosuria, this seldom presents a problem. Specific gravities over 1.020 combined with a high pH may also reduce the sensitivity of the test at low concentrations.[30] By far the greatest source of erroneous glucose results is the technical error of allowing specimens to remain unpreserved at room temperature for extended periods of time. False-negative results will be obtained with both the glucose oxidase and the copper reduction methods due to the rapid glycolysis of glucose.

COPPER REDUCTION TEST

Measurement of glucose by the copper reduction method was one of the earliest chemical tests performed on urine. The test relies on the ability of glucose and other substances to reduce copper sulfate to cuprous oxide in the presence of alkali and heat. A color change progressing from a negative blue through green, yellow, and orange, to brick red occurs when the reaction takes place.

$$CuSO_4 \; (cupric \; ions) + Reducing \; Substance \xrightarrow[\text{alkali}]{\text{heat}}$$
$$Cu_2O \; (cuprous \; ions) + Oxidized \; Substance$$

The classic Benedict's solution was developed in 1908 and contained copper sulfate, sodium carbonate, and sodium citrate buffer.[1] Urine was then added to the solution, heat was applied, and the resulting precipitate was observed for color. A more convenient method that employs Benedict's principle is the Clinitest tablet (Ames Company, Elkhart, Indiana). The tablets contain copper sulfate, sodium carbonate, sodium citrate, and sodium hydroxide. Upon the addition of water and urine, heat is produced by the hydrolysis of sodium hydroxide and its reaction with sodium citrate, and carbon dioxide is released from the sodium carbonate to prevent room air from interfering with the reduction reaction. At the conclusion of the effervescent reaction, a color ranging from blue to orange can be compared against the manufacturer's color chart to determine the approximate amount of glucose present. Care must be taken to observe the reaction closely as it is taking place, because at high glucose levels, a phenomenon known as "pass through" may occur. When this happens, the color produced passes through the orange stage and returns to a blue or blue-green color, and if not observed, a high glucose level may be reported as negative. The manufacturers of Clinitest have suggested a method using two drops instead of five drops of urine to minimize the occurrence of "pass through." However, the ability to detect low levels of glucose may be compromised with the two-drop method, and a separate color chart must be used to interpret the reaction. The original Benedict's test detected very small amounts of glucose, but the sensitivity of Clinitest has been reduced to a minimum level of 200 mg per dl to prevent false-positive reactions from reducing substances, other than glucose, that are present in urine. As a nonspecific test for reducing substances, Clinitest is subject to interference from other reducing sugars, ascorbic acid, certain drug metabolites, and antibiotics such as the cephalosporins. Clinitest tablets are very hygroscopic and should be stored in their tightly closed original bottle. A strong blue color in the unused tablets suggests deterioration due to moisture accumulation, as does vigorous tablet fizzing. Although most laboratories perform the routine urinalysis using dipsticks, many laboratories follow positive glucose results with a Clinitest. All infant urine must be tested by both methods.

COMPARISON OF GLUCOSE OXIDASE AND CLINITEST

Several reasons exist to explain the finding of conflicting results between the two glucose tests. As stated earlier, the Clinitest is not as sensitive as the glucose oxidase test, so the finding of a 1+ dipstick reading and a negative Clinitest should not be surprising. However, a strongly positive dipstick and a negative Clinitest should cause concern about the possible contamination by strong oxidizing agents. The most significant discrepancy is the negative dipstick with a positive Clinitest. Although this may be caused by interfering substances affecting either test, the most frequent cause is the presence of other reducing sugars in the urine. Commonly found sugars include galactose, fructose, pentose, and lactose, of which galactose is the most clinically significant. Galactose in the urine of a newborn represents an inborn error of metabolism in which lack of the enzyme galactose-1-phosphate uridyl transferase prevents breakdown of ingested galactose and results in failure to thrive and other complications, including death. Hospitals should screen all newborns for galactosuria because early detection that results in dietary restriction will control the condition. The appearance of other reducing sugars is usually of minimal clinical significance, and lactose is frequently found in the urine of nursing mothers. Identification is performed using either thin-layer chromatography or the resorcinol test for fructose. Keep in mind that table sugar is sucrose, a nonreducing sugar, and will not react with Clinitest or glucose oxidase strips.

KETONES

The term "ketones" represents three intermediate products of fat metabolism, namely, acetone, acetoacetic acid, and beta-hydroxybutyric acid. Normally, measurable amounts of ketones do not appear in the urine, since all of the metabolized fat is completely broken down into carbon dioxide and water. However, when the use of carbohydrate as the major source of energy becomes compromised, and body stores of fat must be metabolized to supply energy, ketones will be detected in the urine. Clinical reasons for this increased fat metabolism include: the inability to metabolize carbohydrate, as occurs in diabetes mellitus; increased loss of carbohydrate due to vomiting; and inadequate intake of carbohydrate associated with starvation and weight reduction.

CLINICAL SIGNIFICANCE

Testing for urinary ketones is most valuable in the management and monitoring of diabetes mellitus. Ketonuria shows a deficiency in insulin, indicating the need to regulate dosage. It is often an early indicator of insufficient insulin dosage in juvenile diabetes and diabetic patients experiencing medical problems in addition to their diabetes. Increased accumulation of ketones in the blood leads to electrolyte imbalance, dehydration, and if not corrected, acidosis and eventual diabetic coma. To aid in the monitoring of diabetes, ketone tests are not only included in all multiple-test strips, but are also combined with glucose on strips used primarily for at-home testing by diagnosed diabetic patients. The use of multiple-test strips in hospital laboratories will often produce positive ketone tests unrelated to diabetes because the patient's illness is either preventing adequate intake of carbohydrates or is producing an accelerated loss, as in vomiting. A practical application of ketonuria produced by starvation is being used in obesity clinics to determine if patients on high-protein or fasting diets have been cheating.[5]

SUMMARY OF CLINICAL SIGNIFICANCE OF URINE KETONES
1. Diabetic acidosis
2. Insulin dosage monitoring
3. Starvation

DIPSTICK REACTIONS

The three ketone compounds are not present in equal amounts in urine. Both acetone and beta-hydroxybutyric acid are produced from acetoacetic acid, and the proportions of 78 percent beta-hydroxybutyric acid, 20 percent acetoacetic acid, and 2 percent acetone are relatively constant in all specimens.

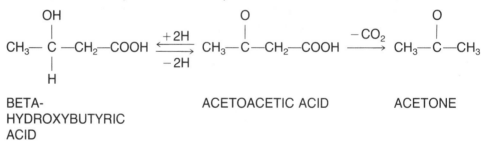

BETA-HYDROXYBUTYRIC ACID   ACETOACETIC ACID   ACETONE

Dipstick tests utilize the sodium nitroprusside reaction to measure ketones. In this reaction, acetoacetic acid in an alkaline medium in the presence of glycine will react with sodium nitroprusside to produce a purple color. The test does not measure beta-hydroxybutyric acid and is only slightly sensitive to acetone; however, since these compounds are derived from acetoacetic acid, their presence can be assumed, and it is not necessary to perform individual tests. Results are reported qualitatively as negative, small, moderate, or large, or as negative, 1+, 2+, or 3+. In cases of severe ketosis, it may be necessary to perform tests on serial dilutions to provide more information as to the degree of ketosis. Acetest (Ames Company, Elkhart, Indiana) provides sodium nitroprusside, glycine, disodium phosphate, and lactose in tablet form. The addition of lactose gives better color differentiation, so the tablet test is often preferred for tests on serial dilutions.

INTERFERING SUBSTANCES

The nitroprusside reaction is subject to a minimum of outside interference. Large concentrations of levodopa may cause false-positive reactions, and specimens collected after diagnostic procedures employing phthalein dyes may produce an interfering red color in the alkaline test medium. The presence of phenylketones in the urine can also distort the color reaction. Improper preservation of specimens will result in falsely decreased values due to the volatilization of acetone and the breakdown of acetoacetic acid by bacteria.[8]

TUBE TESTS

Prior to the introduction of the dipstick and tablet methods, ketones were measured by tube tests. The original nitroprusside test was developed by Legal in 1883; however, a modification by Rothera in 1908 is best known, and the nitroprusside reaction is sometimes referred to as Rothera's test. Tests to measure the individual ketones were also performed and included Gerhardt's test for acetoacetic acid and Hart's test for beta-hydroxybutyric acid. Gerhardt's test combines acetoacetic acid with ferric chloride to produce a red color. Since many compounds, including aspirin, react with ferric chloride, the test is subject to much interference. The removal of acetone and acetoacetic acid by boiling and the reaction of the remaining beta-hydroxybutyric acid with hydrogen peroxide constitute Hart's test. Neither test is considered necessary for clinical evaluation at the present time.

BLOOD

Blood may be present in the urine either in the form of intact red blood cells (hematuria) or as the red blood cell destruction product hemoglobin (hemoglobinuria). As discussed in Chapter 3, blood present in large quantities can be detected visually, with hematuria producing a cloudy red urine and hemoglobinuria appearing as a clear red specimen. However, since any amount of blood greater than three cells per microliter of urine is considered clinically significant, it is not possible to rely on visual examination to detect the presence of blood.[38] Microscopic examination of the urinary sediment will show intact red blood cells; but free hemoglobin, produced either by hemorrhagic disorders or lysis of red blood cells in the urinary tract, will not be detected. Therefore, chemical tests for hemoglobin provide the most accurate means for determining the presence of blood, and once blood has been detected, the microscopic examination can be used to differentiate between hematuria and hemoglobinuria.

CLINICAL SIGNIFICANCE

The finding of hematuria or hemoglobinuria is always considered of major clinical importance and can be associated with numerous pathologic conditions. Hematuria is most closely related to disorders of renal or genitourinary origin in which bleeding is the result of trauma or irritation to the organs of these systems. Major causes of hematuria include renal calculi, glomerulonephritis, tumors, trauma, pyelonephritis, and exposure to toxic chemicals or drugs.[25] The laboratory is frequently requested to perform a urinalysis when patients presenting with severe pain are suspected of having renal calculi, and the finding of hematuria can be essential to the diagnosis. Hemoglobinuria may occur as the result of lysis of red blood cells produced in the urinary tract, or it may be caused by intravascular hemolysis and the subsequent filtering of hemoglobin through the glomerulus. Lysis of red blood cells in the urine will usually show a mixture of hemoglobinuria and hematuria; whereas no red blood cells will be seen in cases of intravascular hemolysis. Under normal conditions, glomerular filtration of hemoglobin is prevented by the formation of large hemoglobin-haptoglobin complexes in the circulation. However, when the amount of free hemoglobin present exceeds the haptoglobin content, as occurs in hemolytic anemias, transfusion reactions, severe burns, infections, and strenuous exercise, hemoglobin is available for glomerular filtration.

SUMMARY OF CLINICAL SIGNIFICANCE OF URINE BLOOD

HEMATURIA

1. Renal calculi
2. Glomerulonephritis
3. Pyelonephritis
4. Tumors
5. Trauma
6. Exposure to toxic chemicals or drugs

HEMOGLOBINURIA

1. Transfusion reactions
2. Hemolytic anemia
3. Severe burns
4. Infections
5. Strenuous exercise

MYOGLOBINURIA

1. Muscular trauma
2. Prolonged coma
3. Convulsions
4. Muscle-wasting diseases
5. Extensive exertion

DIPSTICK REACTIONS

Chemical tests for blood utilize the pseudoperoxidase activity of hemoglobin to catalyze a reaction between hydrogen peroxide and the chromogen o-tolidine to produce oxidized o-tolidine, which has a blue color.

$$H_2O_2 + \text{o-tolidine} \xrightarrow{\substack{\text{hemoglobin} \\ \text{peroxidase}}} \text{Oxidized o-tolidine (blue)} + H_2O$$

Dipstick manufacturers incorporate peroxide, o-tolidine, and buffer into the blood testing area. Two color charts are provided that correspond to the reactions that occur with hemoglobinuria and those seen in hematuria. In the presence of free hemoglobin, uniform color ranging from a negative yellow through green to a strongly positive blue will appear on the pad. In contrast, intact red blood cells are lysed as they come in contact with the pad, and the liberated hemoglobin produces an isolated reaction that results in a speckled pattern on the pad. The degree of hematuria can then be estimated by the intensity of the speckled pattern. Approximate numbers of cells per microliter are supplied by the manufacturers; however, care must be taken when comparing these figures to the actual microscopic values, since the absorbent nature of the pad will attract more than one microliter of urine. The value of the test lies primarily in the ability to differentiate between hemoglobinuria and hematuria and not in the quantitation.

INTERFERING SUBSTANCES

Dipstick tests can detect concentrations between 5 and 10 red blood cells per microliter but are slightly more sensitive to free hemoglobin than to intact red blood cells. High levels of ascorbic acid may produce false-negative results, as will excessive amounts of urinary nitrite associated with severe urinary tract infections. Elevated specific gravity and protein can also reduce the sensitivity of the test. False-positive reactions due to menstrual contamination may be seen, and they will also occur if strong oxidizing detergents are present in the specimen container. False-positive reactions may also be caused by vegetable peroxidase and bacterial enzymes, including an *Escherichia coli* peroxidase. Therefore, sediments containing bacteria should be checked closely for the presence of red blood cells or ghost cells.[42]

MYOGLOBIN

The most well-known interference to the chemical test for blood is the false-positive reaction produced by urinary myoglobin. Myoglobin, a protein found in muscle tissue, not only reacts positively with the chemical test for blood, but also produces a clear red urine. Its presence should be suspected in patients with conditions associated with muscular destruction such as trauma, prolonged coma, convulsions, muscle-wasting diseases, and extensive exertion.[33] Diagnosis of myoglobinuria is usually based on the patient's history and serum tests for enzymes elevated by muscle destruction. The appearance of the patient's serum can sometimes aid in the differentiation between hemoglobinuria and myoglobinuria, since a pink or red serum is seen with hemoglobinuria, and a colorless serum is found in the presence of myoglobin.[2] Specific tests for myoglobin include protein electrophoresis, absorption spectrophotometry, immunodiffusion techniques, and radioimmunoassay.[35] Contamination of urine with povidone-iodine used in surgical procedures will produce a positive chemical test for blood due to the strong oxidizing properties of iodine. If iodine contamination is not suspected, there may be concern that the surgery has caused muscle damage that caused the production of myoglobin.[34]

BILIRUBIN

The appearance of bilirubin in the urine is the first indication of liver disease and is often detected long before the development of jaundice. Bilirubin provides early detection of hepatitis, cirrhosis, gallbladder disease, and cancer, and should be included in every routine urinalysis.[37]

PRODUCTION OF BILIRUBIN

Bilirubin, a highly pigmented yellow compound, is a degradation product of hemoglobin. Under normal conditions, the life span of red blood cells is approximately 120 days, at which time they are destroyed in the spleen and liver by the phagocytic cells of the reticuloendothelial system. The liberated hemoglobin is broken down into its component parts: iron, protein, and protoporphyrin. The iron and protein are reused by the body, and the remaining protoporphyrin is converted to bilirubin by the cells of the reticuloendothelial system. The bilirubin is then released into the circulation, where it binds with albumin and is transported to the liver. At this point, the circulating bilirubin cannot be excreted by the kidneys because not only is it bound to albumin, but it is also water insoluble. In the liver, bilirubin is conjugated with glucuronic acid by the action of glucuronyl transferase to form water-soluble bilirubin diglucuronide. Usually, this conjugated bilirubin will not appear in the urine because it is passed directly from the liver into the bile duct and on to the intestine. In the intestine, it is reduced by intestinal bacteria to urobilinogen and ultimately excreted in the feces in the form of urobilin. Figure 4-1 illustrates bilirubin metabolism for reference with this section and the subsequent discussion of urobilinogen.

CLINICAL SIGNIFICANCE

Conjugated bilirubin will appear in the urine when the normal metabolic cycle is disrupted by obstruction of the bile duct or when the integrity of the liver is damaged,

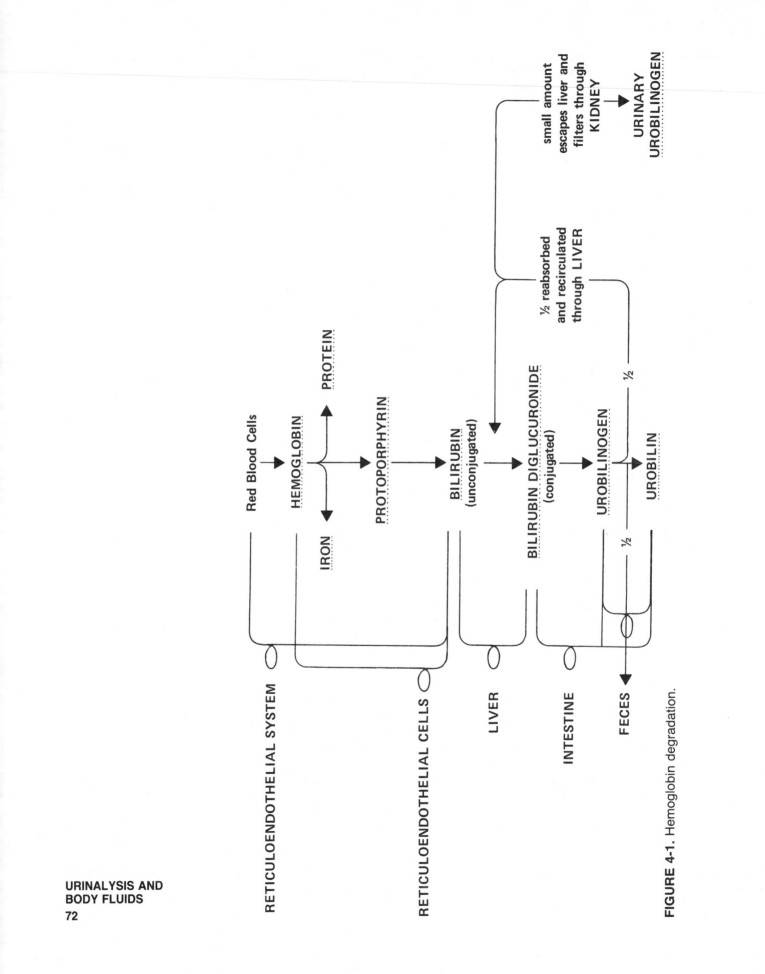

FIGURE 4-1. Hemoglobin degradation.

TABLE 4-3. Urine Bilirubin and Urobilinogen in Jaundice

	Urine Bilirubin	Urine Urobilinogen
Bile duct obstruction	+ + +	Negative
Liver damage	+ or −	+ +
Hemolytic disease	Negative	+ + +

allowing leakage of conjugated bilirubin into the circulation. Hepatitis and cirrhosis are common examples of conditions that produce liver damage resulting in bilirubinuria. Not only does the detection of urinary bilirubin provide an early indication of liver disease, its presence or absence can be used in determining the cause of clinical jaundice. As shown in Table 4-3, this determination can be even more significant when bilirubin results are combined with urinary urobilinogen. Notice that jaundice due to increased destruction of red blood cells does not produce bilirubinuria. This is because the serum bilirubin is present in the unconjugated form and cannot be excreted by the kidney.

SUMMARY OF CLINICAL SIGNIFICANCE OF URINE BILIRUBIN
1. Hepatitis
2. Cirrhosis
3. Biliary obstruction

OXIDATION TESTS
Urine containing bilirubin usually appears dark yellow or amber and produces a yellow foam when shaken. This foam test was actually the first test for bilirubin. A variety of chemical tests based on either oxidation or diazotization reactions are now available. Oxidation tests utilize the ability of ferric chloride dissolved in trichloroacetic acid (Fouchet's reagent) to oxidize bilirubin to biliverdin, producing a green color. The most well known is the Harrison spot test, in which urine mixed with barium sulfate is filtered through heavy filter paper. Bilirubin attached to barium sulfate collects on the filter paper, and the addition of Fouchet's reagent to the dried paper produces a green color. Oxidation tests using ferric chloride are subject to a considerable amount of interference, since many substances, including a metabolite of aspirin, will react with ferric chloride to produce colors that mask the green biliverdin. Highly pigmented urines will also distort the color reaction. Of particular concern are the yellow-orange urines from persons taking Pyridium compounds, since the thick pigment produced may be mistaken for bilirubin on initial examination.

DIPSTICK (DIAZO) REACTIONS
Routine testing for urinary bilirubin by dipstick utilizes the diazo reaction. Bilirubin combines with 2,4-dichloroaniline diazonium salt or 2,6-dichlorobenzene-diazonium-tetra-fluoroborate in an acid medium to produce colors ranging from tan to violet. Qualitative results are reported as negative, small, moderate, or large, or as negative, 1+, 2+, or 3+. Large amounts of ascorbic acid and nitrite may produce false-negative reactions. Dipstick color reactions for bilirubin are more difficult to interpret than other dipstick reactions and are easily influenced by other pigments present in the urine. Even a slight color change should be considered significant because any detectable amount of bilirubin in the urine indicates an abnormal condition.[38] Questionable results should be

retested using the Ictotest (Ames Company, Elkhart, Indiana), which produces a more sharply colored diazo reaction. Ictotest kits consist of testing mats and tablets containing p-nitrobenzene-diazonium-p-toluenesulfonate, sulfosalicylic acid, sodium carbonate, and boric acid. Urine is added to the mat, which has special absorbent properties that cause bilirubin to remain on the surface as the urine filters into the mat. The reagent tablet is then placed on the mat; after water is added, the reaction between the tablet reagents and bilirubin produces a blue or purple color on the surface of the test mat. Colors other than blue or purple appearing on the mat are considered negative. The Ictotest is much more sensitive than the dipstick and is less affected by interfering substances.[9] If interference in the Ictotest is suspected, it can usually be removed by adding water directly to the mat after the urine has been added. Interfering substances will be washed into the mat, and only bilirubin will remain on the surface.

REACTION INTERFERENCE

The false-negative results caused by the testing of specimens that are not fresh are the most frequent errors associated with bilirubin testing. Bilirubin is an unstable compound that is rapidly destroyed when exposed to light. Exposure to room air will cause oxidation of bilirubin to biliverdin, which does not react in the oxidation or diazotization tests. False-negative results will also occur when hydrolysis of bilirubin diglucuronide produces free bilirubin, since this is less reactive in the dipstick tests.[9]

UROBILINOGEN

Like bilirubin, urobilinogen is a bile pigment that results from the degradation of hemoglobin. As shown in Figure 4-1, it is produced in the intestine from the reduction of bilirubin by the intestinal bacteria. Approximately half of the urobilinogen is reabsorbed from the intestine into the blood, recirculates to the liver, and is secreted back into the intestine through the bile duct. The urobilinogen remaining in the intestine is excreted in the feces, where it is oxidized to urobilin, the pigment responsible for the characteristic brown color of the feces. Urobilinogen appears in the urine because, as it circulates in the blood en route to the liver, it passes through the kidney and is filtered by the glomerulus. Therefore, a small amount of urobilinogen, less than 4 mg per 24 hours, is normally found in the urine.

CLINICAL SIGNIFICANCE

Increased urine urobilinogen is seen in liver disease and hemolytic disorders. Impairment of liver function by hepatitis and cirrhosis decreases the liver's ability to process the urobilinogen recirculated from the intestine, and the excess urobilinogen remaining in the blood is filtered by the kidney. Measurement of urine urobilinogen is extremely valuable in the detection of early liver disease, as it is often the only abnormality present.[36] Studies have shown that when urobilinogen tests are performed routinely, 1 percent of a normal population and 9 percent of a hospital population exhibit elevated results.[13] Although the clinical jaundice associated with hemolytic disorders is due to unconjugated bilirubin from the destruction of red blood cells, markedly increased levels of urobilinogen are still seen in the urine. This is because increased amounts of bilirubin are also being conjugated in the liver and passed to the intestine, resulting in increased production of urobilinogen and elevated levels of reabsorbed, circulating urobilinogen. In addition, the overworked liver has difficulty processing the recirculated urobilinogen, so additional amounts are present for urinary excretion. The lack of urobilinogen in the urine and feces is also diagnostically significant and represents an obstruction of the bile duct that prevents the normal passage of bilirubin into the intestine. The relationship of urine urobilinogen and bilirubin to the pathologic conditions associated with them is outlined in Table 4-3.

SUMMARY OF CLINICAL SIGNIFICANCE OF URINE UROBILINOGEN

1. Early detection of liver disease
2. Hemolytic disorders
3. Porphyrinuria

EHRLICH'S TUBE TEST

Until the development of dipstick methods, tests for urobilinogen were not routinely performed because the available procedures were time-consuming and nonspecific. The reagent used in all tests was p-dimethylaminobenzaldehyde (Ehrlich's reagent). Addition of Ehrlich's reagent to urine containing urobilinogen produces a cherry red color; however, other substances found in urine and referred to as Ehrlich-reactive compounds will also produce a positive reaction. These include porphobilinogen, indican, p-aminosalicylic acid, and sulfonamides. To produce a semiquantitative measurement, the original method of adding Ehrlich's reagent to urine and observing against a white background for the presence of a red color was modified to test serial dilutions of urine. Positive results in dilutions greater than 1 to 20 were considered significant. To avoid missing the presence of a faint pink color in higher dilutions, it was recommended that tubes be examined by looking down through the top while holding the bottom against a white background. A more precise method was developed by Watson in which the intensity of the red color was measured spectrophotometrically. Sodium acetate was also added to enhance the reaction and to make it more specific. Results obtained with any method using Ehrlich's reagent are reported in Ehrlich units. An Ehrlich unit is essentially equal to 1 mg of urobilinogen, but may contain a proportionate amount of Ehrlich-reactive compounds. Since most interfering substances increase proportionately with urobilinogen, an increase in Ehrlich units can be considered to represent an increase in urobilinogen.[44] Normal values for females are 0.1 to 1.1 Ehrlich units and for males are 0.3 to 2.1 Ehrlich units. These values are based on the recommended 2-hour specimen collected between 2 and 4 PM, which is believed to be the time of greatest urobilinogen excretion.[40] Improper collection and preservation of specimens produce the most frequent errors in urobilinogen testing. Due to the light sensitivity of urobilinogen, specimens should be tested immediately or stored in a dark container. False-negative results may also be reported from random specimens, as the largest amounts of urobilinogen are excreted within 2 to 3 hours after meals.[44]

WATSON-SCHWARTZ DIFFERENTIATION TEST

Although the presence of most Ehrlich-reactive compounds is not considered important, urinary porphobilinogen is pathologically significant and will be discussed in Chapter 6. The classic test for differentiating between urobilinogen and porphobilinogen is the Watson-Schwartz test.[41] After production of the cherry red color using sodium acetate and Ehrlich's reagent, the specimen is divided into two tubes. The addition of chloroform to one tube will result in the extraction of urobilinogen into the chloroform layer, producing a colorless top urine layer with a red chloroform layer on the bottom. Neither porphobilinogen nor other Ehrlich-reactive compounds are soluble in chloroform. Porphobilinogen is also not soluble in butanol; however, urobilinogen and other Ehrlich-reactive compounds will be extracted into butanol. Therefore, the addition of butanol to the second tube will produce a red upper (butanol) layer if urobilinogen or Ehrlich-reactive compounds are present and a colorless butanol layer if porphobilinogen is present. As summarized in Figure 4-2, urobilinogen is soluble in both chloroform and

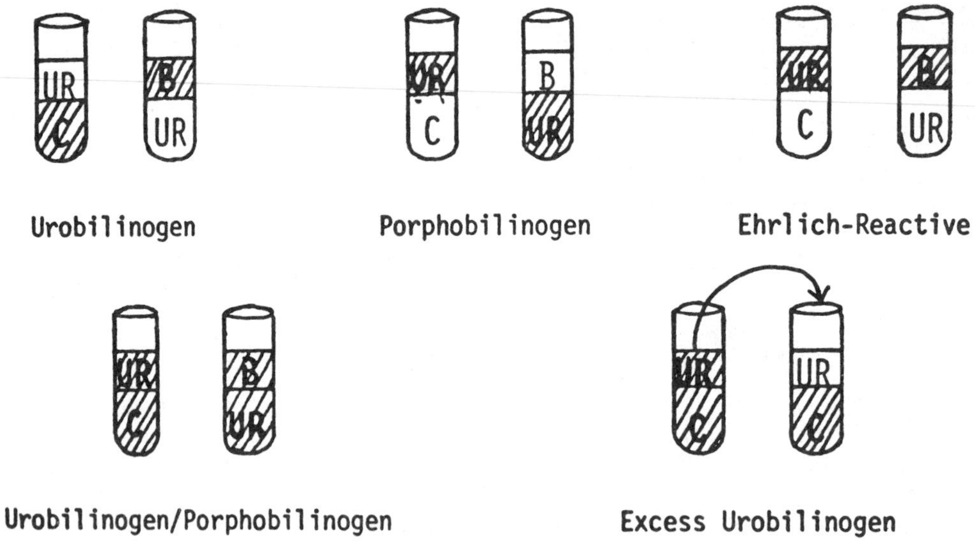

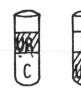
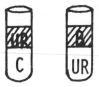

Urobilinogen   Porphobilinogen   Ehrlich-Reactive

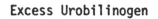

Urobilinogen/Porphobilinogen   Excess Urobilinogen

FIGURE 4-2. Typical Ehrlich reactions. (Adapted from Bradley and Schumann,[2] p. 411.)

butanol, and porphobilinogen is soluble in neither. If both urobilinogen and porphobilinogen are present, both layers will appear red. However, before reporting the test as positive for both substances, an additional chloroform extraction should be performed on the red urine layer to ensure that the red color is not due to excess urobilinogen.

DIPSTICK REACTIONS AND INTERFERENCE

Until recently, dipstick tests for urobilinogen utilized *p*-dimethylaminobenzaldehyde reacting in an acid medium to produce colors ranging from tan to orange. As with the tube tests, this method is also subject to interference by Ehrlich-reacting compounds. Use of 4-methoxybenzene-diazonium-tetrafluoroborate by Chemstrip has produced a more specific test, with colors ranging from pink to red. False-negative results may occur when large quantities of nitrite are present, and highly pigmented urine may obscure the color reactions. However, there is no interference from the Ehrlich-reactive substances. Both tests will detect urobilinogen present in normal quantities, and color comparisons are provided for the upper limits of normal as well as abnormal concentrations. Dipstick tests cannot determine the absence of urobilinogen, which is significant in biliary obstruction.

NITRITE
CLINICAL SIGNIFICANCE

The dipstick test for nitrite provides a rapid screening test for the presence of urinary tract infection. It is not designed to replace the urine culture as the primary test for diagnosing and monitoring bacterial infection, but instead to detect those cases in which the need for a culture may not be apparent. Urinary tract infections are seen most frequently in women, young children, and the elderly.[22] The majority of infections are believed to start in the bladder as a result of external contamination and, if untreated, progress upward through the ureters to the tubules, renal pelvis, and kidney. The nitrite test is valuable for detecting initial bladder infection (cystitis), since patients are often asymptomatic or have vague symptoms that would not lead the physician to order a urine culture. Pyelonephritis, an inflammatory process of the kidney and adjacent renal pelvis, is a frequent complication of untreated cystitis and can lead to renal tissue damage, impairment of renal function, hypertension, and even septicemia.[22] Therefore, detection of bacteriuria through the use of the nitrite screening test, and subsequent antibiotic therapy, can prevent these serious complications from developing. The nitrite test can also be used to evaluate the success of antibiotic therapy and to periodically screen persons with recurrent infections or diabetics and pregnant women, who are considered to be at high risk for urinary tract infection.[23]

SUMMARY OF CLINICAL SIGNIFICANCE OF URINE NITRITE
1. Cystitis
2. Pyelonephritis
3. Evaluation of antibiotic therapy
4. Monitoring of patients at high risk for urinary tract infection
5. Screening of urine culture specimens

DIPSTICK REACTIONS
The chemical basis of the nitrite test is the ability of certain bacteria to reduce nitrate, a normal constituent of urine, to nitrite, which does not normally appear in the urine. Nitrite is detected by the Griess reaction, in which nitrite at an acidic pH reacts with an aromatic amine (para-arsanilic acid or sulfanilamide) to form a diazonium compound that then reacts with 3-hydroxy-1,2,3,4-tetrahydrobenz-(h)-quinolin to produce a pink color. To prevent false-positive reactions due to externally contaminated specimens, the sensitivity of the test is standardized to correspond with the bacterial culture criteria that require a positive urine specimen to contain 100,000 organisms per milliliter. Although different shades of pink may be produced, the test does not measure the degree of bacteriuria, and any shade of pink is considered to represent a clinically significant amount of bacteria.

REACTION INTERFERENCE
Several major factors can influence the reliability of the nitrite test, and negative tests in the presence of even vaguely suspicious clinical symptoms should always be repeated or followed by a urine culture. The ability to reduce nitrate to nitrite is not possessed by all bacteria, although it is found in the gram-negative bacteria that most frequently cause urinary tract infections. However, a significant number of infections are caused by non–nitrate-reducing gram-positive bacteria and yeasts, and the presence of these organisms will not be detected by the nitrite test. Bacteria capable of reducing nitrate must also remain in contact with the urinary nitrate long enough to produce nitrite. Therefore, it is recommended that all nitrite tests be performed on first morning specimens because urine will have been held in the bladder for several hours. The correlation between positive cultures and positive nitrite tests is significantly lower when testing is perfomed on random samples.[26] Likewise, it is imperative to perform nitrite testing on fresh urine samples, because multiplication of contaminant bacteria will soon produce measurable amounts of nitrite. When fresh urine is tested, false-positive results will not be obtained even if the specimen is collected in a nonsterile container. The reliability of the test is also dependent on the presence of adequate amounts of nitrate in the urine. This is seldom a problem in patients on a normal diet that contains green vegetables; however, since diet is not usually controlled prior to testing, the possibility of a false-negative result due to lack of dietary nitrate does exist. Other sources of false-negative tests include inhibition of bacterial metabolism by antibiotics, the presence of large amounts of ascorbic acid, and the further reduction of nitrite to nondetectable nitrogen, which may occur when large numbers of bacteria are present.

SPECIFIC GRAVITY
The recent addition of a specific gravity testing area to Multistix has eliminated a time-consuming step in the routine urinalysis and has provided a convenient way to closely monitor patient hydration in areas that must analyze small quantities of urine.[14]

DIPSTICK REACTION

The test is based on the change in pK (dissociation constant) of poly (methyl vinyl ether-maleic anhydride). The polyelectrolyte ionizes in proportion to the ions in solution, producing a change in pH that is detected by the indicator bromthymol blue.[7] As specific gravity increases, bromthymol blue changes from blue-green to green and finally to yellow-green. Readings between 1.000 and 1.030 can be made at 0.005 intervals by careful comparison with the color chart.

REACTION INTERFERENCE

Urine pH of 6.5 or over may interfere with the reaction because bromthymol blue is active in this range. Therefore, it is recommended that 0.005 be added to the specific gravity readings from urines in this pH range.[7] Unlike the physical methods for measuring specific gravity, the chemical method is not affected by glucose, protein, or radiographic dyes.[18] Good correlation has been shown between the chemical method and corrected urinometer and refractometer readings.[4]

SUMMARY OF CLINICAL SIGNIFICANCE OF URINE SPECIFIC GRAVITY

1. Patient hydration and dehydration
2. Loss of renal tubular concentrating ability
3. Diabetes insipidus
4. Determination of unsatisfactory specimens due to low concentration.

LEUKOCYTES

A new development in dipstick testing is the Chemstrip-L (Bio-Dynamics/BMC, Indianapolis, Indiana) for the detection of urinary leukocytes. One of the most frequent findings in the routine urinalysis is the presence of leukocytes, which indicates a possible infection of the urinary tract. Detection of leukocytes was previously made only by microscopic examination of the urinary sediment. This can be subject to variation depending on the method used to prepare the sediment and the technical personnel examining the sediment. Therefore, the chemical test for leukocytes offers a more standardized means for the detection of leukocytes.[24] The test is not designed to measure the concentration of leukocytes, and the manufacturer recommends that quantitation be done by microscopic examination.

SUMMARY OF CLINICAL SIGNIFICANCE OF URINE LEUKOCYTES

1. Urinary tract infection
2. Screening of urine culture specimens

DIPSTICK REACTION

The chemical reaction is enzymatic, using the esterases present in granulocytic white blood cells to convert indoxyl carboxylic acid ester to indoxyl, which is subsequently oxidized by room air to indigo blue.

$$\text{Indoxyl Carboxylic Acid Ester} \xrightarrow{\text{esterases}} \text{Indoxyl} \xrightarrow{\text{oxidation}} \text{Indigo Blue}$$

To obtain optimum color production, the initial strips had to remain exposed to room air for 15 minutes before being compared with the color chart. The time of the leukocyte reaction has been shortened on the Chemstrip-9 dipsticks by the addition of a diazonium salt to the test pad. Reaction of indigo blue with the diazonium salt produces a purple color within 2 minutes. The color chart contains four areas representing negative, trace, 1+, and 2+. It is recommended that trace reactions be repeated on a fresh specimen and that microscopic examinations be performed on all positive specimens. The Chemstrip LN (leukocyte and nitrite) can be used to screen specimens prior to performing a culture and provides a negative predictive value of 95.6 percent and considerable cost reduction.[43]

REACTION INTERFERENCE

Other than the presence of strong oxidizing agents in the collection container, no causes of false-positive reactions have been found. Erythrocytes, bacteria, and renal tissue cells do not contain esterases. False-negative results may occur in the presence of high levels of ascorbic acid and protein. Urines with a large amount of yellow pigment may produce a green instead of a blue color, and this should be interpreted as a positive reaction. An additional advantage to the chemical leukocyte test is that it will detect the presence of leukocytes that have been lysed and would not appear in the microscopic examination.[10]

REFERENCES

1. BENEDICT, SR: *A reagent for the detection of reducing sugars.* J Biol Chem 5:485–487, 1909.
2. BRADLEY, M AND SCHUMANN, BB: *Examination of the urine.* In HENRY, JB (ED): *Clinical Diagnosis and Management by Laboratory Methods.* WB Saunders, Philadelphia, 1984.
3. BRERETON, DM, SONTOP, ME, AND FRASER, CG: *Timing of urinalysis reactions when reagent strips are used.* Clin Chem 24(8):1420–1421, 1978.
4. BURKHARDT, AE, ET AL: *A reagent strip for measuring the specific gravity of urine.* Clin Chem 28(10):2068–2072, 1981.
5. DRENICK, EJ: *Weight reduction with low calorie diets.* JAMA 202(2):136–138, 1967.
6. FELDMAN, JR, KELLEY, WN, AND LEBOVITZ, HE: *Inhibition of glucose oxidase paper tests by reducing metabolites.* Diabetes 19(5):337–343, 1970.
7. FREE, AH: *A colourimetric method for urine specific gravity compared with current direct and indirect procedures.* Br J Clin Prac 36(9):307–311, 1982.
8. FREE, AH AND FREE, HM: *Nature of nitroprusside reactive material in urine ketosis.* Am J Clin Pathol 30(1):7–10, 1958.
9. FREE, AH AND FREE, HM: *Urodynamics: Concepts Relating to Routine Urine Chemistry.* Ames Division, Miles Laboratories, Elkhart, Indiana, 1978.
10. GILLENWATER, JY: *Detection of urinary leukocytes by Chemstrip-L.* J Urol 125:383–384, 1981.
11. GUTHRIE, D, HINNEN, D, AND GUTHRIE, R: *Single-voided vs. double-voided urine testing.* Diabetes Care 2(3):269–271, 1979.
12. GYURE, W: *Comparison of several methods for semiquantitative determination of urinary protein.* Clin Chem 23(5):876–879, 1977.
13. HAGER, CB AND FREE, AH: *Urine urobilinogen as a component of routine urinalysis.* Am J Med Technol 36(5):227–233, 1970.
14. HENSEY, OJ AND COOKE, RWI: *Estimation of urine specific gravity and osmolarity using a simple reagent strip.* Br Med J 286(6358):53, 1983.
15. HOELTGE, GA AND ERSTS, A: *A quality control system for the general urinalysis laboratory.* Am J Clin Pathol 73(3):404–408, 1980.
16. JAMES, GP, BEE, DE, AND FULLER, JB: *Accuracy and precision of urinary pH determinations using two commercially available dipsticks.* Am J Clin Pathol 70(3):368–374, 1978.

17. KARK, RM, ET AL: *A Primer of Urinalysis.* Harper & Row, New York, 1963.
18. KAVELMAN, DA: *A representative of Ames responds.* Clin Chem 29(1):210–211, 1983.
19. KILLINGSWORTH, LM, COONEY, SK, AND TYLLIA, MM: *Protein analysis: Finding clues to disease in the urine.* Diagnostic Medicine 3(3):69–75, 1980.
20. KINNEY, AB AND BLOUNT, M: *Effect of cranberry juice on urinary pH.* Nurs Res 28(5):287–290, 1979.
21. KOLTHOFF, I: *Acid-Base Indicators.* Macmillan, New York, 1937.
22. KUNIN, CM: *Prevention and Management of Urinary Tract Infections.* Lea & Febiger, Philadelphia, 1979.
23. KUNIN, CM AND DEGROOT, JE: *Self-screening for significant bacteriuria.* JAMA 231(13):1349–1353, 1975.
24. KUSUMI, RK, GROVER, PJ, AND KUNIN, CM: *Rapid detection of pyuria by leukocyte esterase activity.* JAMA 245(16):1653–1655, 1981.
25. LEONARDO, JR: *Simple test for hematuria compared with established tests.* JAMA 179(10):807–808, 1962.
26. MONTE-VERDE, D AND NOSANCHUK, JS: *The sensitivity and specificity of nitrite testing for bacteriuria.* Laboratory Medicine 12(12):755–757, 1981.
27. PARVING, H, ET AL: *Early detection of patients at risk of developing diabetic neuropathy: A longitudinal study of urinary albumin excretion.* Acta Endocrinol 100(4):550–555, 1982.
28. PEELE, JD, GADSDEN, RH, AND CREWS, R: *Semi-automated vs. visual reading of urinalysis dipsticks.* Clin Chem 23(12):2242–2246, 1977.
29. PEELE, JD, GADSDEN, RH, AND CREWS, R: *Evaluation of Ames' "Clini-Tek."* Clin Chem 23(12):2238–2241, 1977.
30. *Product Profile: N-Multistix, Reagent Strips for Urinalysis.* Ames Division, Miles Laboratories, Elkhart, Indiana, 1980.
31. RACE, GJ AND WHITE, MG: *Basic Urinalysis.* Harper & Row, Hagerstown, Maryland, 1979.
32. RAUBER, AP AND MARONCELLI, RD: *Effects of dietary changes on alkalinization of urine pH.* Vet Hum Toxicol (Suppl) 23:46–47, 1981.
33. ROWLAND, LP AND PENN, AS: *Myoglobinuria.* Med Clin North Am 56(6):1233–1256, 1972.
34. SAID, R: *Contamination of urine with povidone-iodine: Cause of false-positive test for occult blood in urine.* JAMA 242(8):748–749, 1979.
35. SARANCHAK, HJ AND BERNSTEIN, SH: *A new diagnostic test for acute myocardial infarction: The detection of myoglobinuria by radioimmunodiffusion assay.* JAMA 228(10):1251–1255, 1974.
36. SHERLOCK, S: *Diseases of the Liver and Biliary System.* FA Davis, Philadelphia, 1965.
37. SHUTKINS, MW AND CAINE, D: *The clinical value of bilirubin determinations in routine urinalysis with an improved method.* Am J Gastroenterol 23(3):235–240, 1955.
38. *Urinalysis with Chemstrip.* Bio-Dynamics, Division of Boehringer Mannheim, Indianapolis, Indiana, 1978.
39. VIBERTI, GC AND VERGANI, D: *Detection of potentially reversible diabetic albuminuria: A three-drop agglutination test for urinary albumin at low concentration.* Diabetes 31(11):973–975, 1982.
40. WATSON, CJ, ET AL: *Studies of urobilinogen. V. A simple method for the quantitative recording of the Ehrlich reaction as carried out with urine and feces.* Am J Clin Pathol 14:605–615, 1944.
41. WATSON, CJ AND SCHWARTZ, S: *A simple test for urinary porphobilinogen.* Proc Soc Exp Biol Med 47:393–394, 1941.
42. WEAVER, MR AND GIBB, I: *Urinalysis for blood: Questionable interpretation of reagent strip results.* Clin Chem 29(2):401–402, 1983.

43. WISE, KA, SAGERT, LA, AND GRAMMENS, GL: *Urine leukocyte esterase and nitrite tests as an aid to predict urine culture results.* Laboratory Medicine 15(3):186–187, 1984.
44. WITH, T: *Bile Pigments.* Academic Press, New York, 1968.

STUDY QUESTIONS (Choose one best answer)

1. Proper care of dipsticks used for urine chemical tests includes all of the following except:

   a. checking the expiration date
   b. storing in the refrigerator
   c. preventing exposure to volatile fumes
   d. storing with desiccant

2. The reactivity of dipsticks should be checked

       1. during each laboratory shift
       2. when a new bottle is opened
       3. using positive controls
       4. using positive and negative controls
       5. when pads appear discolored
   a. 1, 2, and 3
   b. 3 and 5
   c. 1, 2, and 4
   d. 2 only

3. A urine specimen with a pH of 9.0 would indicate that the patient should be:

   a. tested further for metabolic or respiratory alkalosis
   b. changed to a diet high in cranberry juice to lower the pH
   c. asked to collect a fresh specimen for immediate testing
   d. placed on medication to lower the pH

4. To produce pH readings at intervals between 5 and 9, dipsticks must use a:

   a. broad-range indicator
   b. narrow-range, broad-spectrum indicator
   c. combination of two low-range and two high-range indicators
   d. double-indicator system

5. A patient has a 1 + protein reaction on a specimen collected in the doctor's office. The doctor instructs the patient to go home and rest and to collect a specimen immediately upon arising the next day. The second specimen is negative for protein. This indicates:

   a. nocturnal proteinuria
   b. orthostatic proteinuria
   c. Bence Jones proteinuria
   d. diurnal proteinuria

6. The principle of the dipstick reaction for protein is based on:

   a. protein producing an error in the color of an indicator at pH 3.
   b. protein being oxidized by an enzymatic reaction
   c. protein reacting with sulfosalicylic acid on the reagent pad
   d. protein producing a change in pH that is detected by an indicator on the reagent pad

7. False-positive dipstick reactions for protein will occur with all of the following except:

   a. strongly alkaline urines
   b. quaternary ammonium compounds
   c. loss of buffer from the reagent pad
   d. high salt concentrations

8. Bence Jones protein excreted in the urine in cases of multiple myeloma has a unique characteristic of:

   a. reacting with dipsticks and not sulfosalicylic acid
   b. precipitating with acetic acid and heat and not with sulfosalicylic acid
   c. precipitating when heated to 60°C and dissolving at 100°C
   d. precipitating when heated to 100°C and dissolving when cooled to 60°C

9. Clinical conditions associated with glycosuria include:

   1. diabetes mellitus
   2. diabetes insipidus
   3. renal tubular damage
   4. head injuries
   a. 1 only
   b. 1, 2, and 3
   c. 1 and 3
   d. 1, 3, and 4

10. Dipstick tests for glucose utilize:

    a. double sequential enzyme reactions
    b. copper reduction
    c. peroxidase activity of glucose
    d. buffered reaction of mixed enzyme indicators

11. Which of the following statements is (are) correct for glucose testing by dipstick?

    1. glucose oxidase reacts with glucose in the urine
    2. non–glucose-reducing substances fail to react
    3. ascorbic acid may cause a false-negative reaction
    4. hydrogen peroxide and peroxidase react to oxidize a chromogen
    a. 1 only
    b. 1, 2, and 3
    c. 1, 2, and 4
    d. 1, 2, 3, and 4

12. Galactose will:

    a. react with Multistix but not Clinitest
    b. react with Multistix but not Chemstrip

c. react with Multistix and Chemstrip
d. react with Clinitest but not Chemstrip

13. While performing a Clinitest, you observe that the color changes rapidly from blue to orange and then back to blue. You should:

    a. report the test as negative since the final reaction color is blue
    b. report the test as negative because the brief orange color probably was from detergent in the tube
    c. repeat the test using fewer drops of urine or diluted urine to check for "pass through"
    d. repeat the test using more drops of urine to prevent "pass through"

14. A 1+ dipstick reaction and a 4+ Clinitest reaction could indicate the:

    a. presence of glucose and other reducing substances
    b. presence of glucose only
    c. presence of non–glucose-reducing substances only
    d. presence of contamination by a strong oxidizing agent

15. In the routine urinalysis, the term ketones refers to all of the following except:

    a. acetone
    b. acetoacetic acid
    c. phenylketones
    d. beta-hydroxybutyric acid

16. Ketosis is most frequently associated with:

    a. diabetes insipidus
    b. diabetes mellitus
    c. phenylketonuria
    d. metabolic alkalosis

17. Dipstick tests for ketones react most strongly with:

    a. acetone
    b. acetoacetic acid
    c. phenylketones
    d. beta-hydroxybutyric acid

18. The finding of a 2+ dipstick reaction for blood in the urine of a patient with severe lower back pain can aid in confirming a diagnosis of:

    a. pyelonephritis
    b. appendicitis
    c. renal calculi
    d. multiple myeloma

19. A clear red urine with a 4+ dipstick reaction for blood may contain:

    a. hemoglobin
    b. lysed red blood cells
    c. myoglobin
    d. all of the above

20. Dipstick reactions for blood are based on the:

  a. oxidation of hemoglobin peroxidase
  b. reaction of hemoglobin with ortho-tolidine
  c. peroxidase activity of hemoglobin
  d. detection of a pH change introduced by the presence of hemoglobin

21. A urinalysis report shows:

urobilinogen	4 EU
bilirubin	negative
blood	small
nitrite	negative

  This suggests:
  a. abnormal destruction of RBCs in the body
  b. inflammation of the liver
  c. severe upper urinary tract infection
  d. a normal urine specimen

22. The principle of the dipstick test for bilirubin is:

  a. bilirubin causes a color change when it binds to a buffered pH indicator
  b. bilirubin binds to a diazonium salt to form a colored complex
  c. bilirubin is oxidized to biliverdin
  d. bilirubin causes a pH change detected by the reagent pad indicator

23. A yellow foam observed after shaking a greenish amber urine indicates that the:

  a. urine may contain sulfa crystals
  b. patient may have hemolytic jaundice
  c. urine may contain bilirubin
  d. urine should be tested with Ictotest for the presence of urobilinogen

24. A positive urine bilirubin with a negative test for urobilinogen indicates:

  a. intravascular hemolysis
  b. biliary duct obstruction
  c. hepatitis
  d. cirrhosis

25. The ideal specimen for urobilinogen testing is:

  a. collected over 24 hours and preserved with hydrochloric acid
  b. collected between 2 and 4 in the afternoon and preserved with hydrochloric acid
  c. collected over 24 hours in a dark bottle
  d. collected between 2 and 4 in the afternoon in a dark bottle

26. Ehrlich's reagent contains:

  a. tetrabromphenol blue
  b. para-hydroxybutyrate
  c. para-dimethylaminobenzaldehyde
  d. dichloroaniline diazonium salt

27. A specimen that produces a cherry red color is extracted with chloroform and

butanol. If the positive reaction is caused by porphobilinogen, you would expect the extraction to show:

a. extraction into chloroform and butanol
b. extraction into chloroform but not butanol
c. extraction into butanol but not chloroform
d. no extraction into chloroform or butanol

28. A specimen that produces a cherry red color with Ehrlich's reagent is extracted into chloroform and both the aqueous and chloroform layers are red. You should:

a. repeat the test with chloroform from a new bottle
b. extract the aqueous layer into more chloroform
c. extract the specimen into butanol
d. report the presence of both urobilinogen and porphobilinogen

29. The dipstick nitrite test is based on:

a. the utilization of nitrite by bacteria present in the urine
b. the reaction of nitrite with the cell wall of gram-negative bacteria
c. the reduction of nitrate in urine to nitrite by bacteria
d. the reaction of bacterial nitrite with an aromatic amine to produce a pH change

30. All of the following can cause false-negative nitrite tests in the presence of significant bacteriuria except:

a. performing the test on urine that has remained in the bladder for several hours
b. inadequate ingestion of dietary nitrate supplemented with vitamin C
c. performing the test on a random clean-catch specimen
d. production of nitrogen from the presence of large numbers of bacteria

31. The principle of the dipstick test for specific gravity is:

a. ionization of the indicator bromthymol blue, producing a pH change
b. ionization of a polyelectrolyte, producing a pH change
c. reaction of dissociated polyelectrolyte with bromthymol blue to produce a pH change
d. change in the pK of bromthymol blue to produce a pH change

32. Major advantages of the leukocyte esterase dipstick test include all of the following except:

a. it will detect the presence of lysed leukocytes
b. it can be used to screen specimens prior to bacterial culturing
c. it is a more standardized method for detecting leukocytes than the microscopic method
d. it will accurately quantitate the leukocytes present

33. What do the following results suggest?

Color: yellow, hazy	Bilirubin: negative
Sp. Gr.: 1.019	Urobilinogen: 0.1 EU
pH: 8	Blood: negative
Glucose: negative	Nitrite: positive
Protein: trace	Leukocytes: positive
Ketone: negative	

a. diabetes mellitus
b. unsatisfactory specimen
c. urinary tract infection
d. normal female specimen

34. Matching (Indicate which substance is measured with the listed reagents. NOTE: Some substances may be used more than once.)

_____ tetrabromphenol	a. blood
_____ nitroprusside and an alkaline buffer	b. bilirubin
_____ *o*-tolidine	c. protein
_____ sulfosalicylic acid	d. urobilinogen
_____ NaCl + acetic acid	e. ketone
_____ *p*-dimethylaminobenzaldehyde	f. glucose
_____ methyl red and bromthymol blue	g. pH
_____ 2,6-dichlorobenzene-diazonium-tetrafluoroborate	
_____ copper sulfate + sodium hydroxide	
_____ barium chloride + Fouchet's reagent	

35. Analysis of a urine specimen produces the following results:

Color: dark yellow   Ketone: moderate
Appearance: clear   Bilirubin: negative
Sp. Gr.: 1.028   Urobilinogen: 0.1 EU
pH: 5.0   Nitrite: negative
Protein: negative   Leukocytes: negative
Glucose: negative

Determine whether or not each of the following patients would be expected to produce the urine:
a. a 7-year-old girl with uncontrolled diarrhea and vomiting for 3 days
b. an uncontrolled diabetic patient 2 hours postprandial
c. a 25-year-old woman on a low-carbohydrate, high-protein diet
d. a 42-year-old man on diuretics with adequate fluid intake

36. A 20-year-old female vegetarian who supplements her diet with megavitamins visits her doctor complaining of back pain and frequent painful urination. A urinalysis shows the following:

Color: amber   Blood: moderate
Appearance: cloudy   Ketone: negative
Sp. Gr.: 1.010   Bilirubin: negative
pH: 8.0   Urobilinogen: 0.1 EU
Protein: 2+   Nitrite: negative
Glucose: negative   Leukocytes: trace

a. Knowing the patient's clinical symptoms, do you find any discrepancies in the results? Explain your answer.
b. Could the presence of blood be contributing to the 2+ protein reading? Why?
c. What could explain the discrepancy between the patient's urine color, specific gravity, and frequent urination?
d. Give two reasons that could account for the high pH on this freshly voided specimen.

5
MICROSCOPIC EXAMINATION OF THE URINE

INSTRUCTIONAL OBJECTIVES

Upon completion of this chapter, readers will be able to:

1. list eight formed elements found in urinary sediments

2. discuss the methods used by commercial systems to standardize the microscopic examination

3. name the four elements measured in the Addis count and recognize their normal values

4. describe the eight standard steps for performing the microscopic urinalysis

5. distinguish between relative centrifugal force and revolutions per minute

6. correlate physical and chemical urinalysis results with microscopic observations

7. name the dyes used in the Sternheimer-Malbin and Sternheimer stains

8. describe "glitter cells" and discuss their origin

9. differentiate among phase-contrast, interference-contrast, and polarized microscopy

10. list the normal values for red blood cells, white blood cells, and hyaline casts

11. discuss the significance of red blood cells in the urinary sediment

12. differentiate among red blood cells, yeast, and oil droplets

13. discuss the significance of white blood cells in the urinary sediment

14. name, describe, and give the origin of the three types of epithelial cells found in the urinary sediment

15. differentiate between leukocytes and renal tubular epithelial cells

16. discuss the significance of oval fat bodies

17. list four conditions necessary for urinary cast formation

18. name the major protein found in casts

19. discuss the significance of hyaline, red blood cell, white blood cell, epithelial cell, granular, waxy, and fatty casts

20. explain why the appearance of broad casts may indicate serious renal disease

21. explain the importance of identifying urinary crystals

22. list and describe the normal crystals found in acidic urine

23. list and describe the normal crystals found in alkaline urine

24. describe and state the significance of cystine, cholesterol, leucine, tyrosine, sulfonamide, radiographic dye, and ampicillin crystals

25. discuss the procedures and documentation for quality control of specimens, methodology, reagents, control materials, instrumentation, equipment, and reporting of results in the urinalysis laboratory

HISTORY AND SIGNIFICANCE

The third part of the routine urinalysis is the microscopic examination of the urinary sediment. Its purpose is to detect and identify insoluble materials present in the urine. The blood, kidney, lower genitourinary tract, and external contamination all contribute formed elements to the urine. These include red and white blood cells, casts, epithelial cells, bacteria, yeast, parasites, mucus, spermatozoa, crystals, and artifacts. Because some of these components are of no clinical significance and others are considered normal unless they are present in increased amounts, examination of the urinary sediment must include both identification and quantitation of the elements present.

The urine microscopic examination is the least standardized and most time-consuming part of the routine urinalysis. Its value has been controversial since 1936, when the well-known renal specialist, Dr. Henry Christians, stated that "it is impossible to diagnose accurately during life the anatomical changes in the kidney that will be found after death."[19] Interest in the urine microscopic has lagged behind other urine tests ever since that time, even though it is now known that careful analysis of the sediment components can provide early information concerning the anatomic integrity of the kidney and the existence and extent of renal damage.[28]

While significant advances have been made in the methodology, sensitivity, and specificity of the urine chemistry tests, the microscopic lacks standardization, adequate quality control, and automation. Studies have been done to determine the advantages of performing the microscopic on routine specimens that have normal physical and chemical results. Percentages of abnormal specimens that would go undetected vary greatly among the studies.[29,35] The development of a chemical test for leukocytes has also decreased the number of abnormalities that would be overlooked if no microscopic examination is performed, particularly if specimens are midstream clean-catches.[2,25,32] However, whether it remains a part of the routine urinalysis or not, the microscopic is still a valuable diagnostic aid. Efforts are underway to improve its reliability through standardized techniques, improved quality control, and continuing education of technical personnel.

METHODOLOGY

The microscopic analysis is subject to several procedural variations, including methods by which the sediment is prepared, amounts of sediment actually examined, methods and equipment used to obtain visualization, and the manner in which results are reported. A procedure to quantitate formed elements in the urine microscopic was developed by Addis in 1926. The Addis count, as it is called, used a hemocytometer to count the number of red and white blood cells, casts, and epithelial cells present in a 12-hour specimen. Normal values have a wide range and are approximately 0 to 500,000 red blood cells, 0 to 1,800,000 white blood cells and epithelial cells, and 0 to 5,000 hyaline casts.[1] The Addis count was used primarily to monitor the course of diagnosed cases of renal disease. It is seldom used today because commercial systems such as the KOVA (ICL Scientific, Fountain Valley, California) and the T-System (Whale Scientific, Inc., Commerce City, Colorado) are available to provide standardization of the microscopic procedure. Whether or not a laboratory chooses to adopt a commercial system, the following similar methodology is recommended:

1. Specimens should be examined while fresh or adequately preserved. Formed elements, primarily red and white blood cells and hyaline casts, disintegrate rapidly, particularly in dilute alkaline urine.
2. A standard amount of urine, usually between 10 and 15 ml, is centrifuged in a conical tube. This will provide an adequate volume from which to obtain a representative sample of the elements present in the specimen.
3. The speed of the centrifuge and the length of time the specimen is centrifuged should be consistent. Centrifugation for 5 minutes at a relative centrifugal force (RCF) of 400 will produce an optimum amount of sediment with the least chance of damaging the elements. To correct for differences in the diameter of centrifuge heads, the RCF rather than the RPM (revolutions per minute) is used. The RPM value shown on the centrifuge tachometer can be converted to RCF using nomograms available in many laboratory manuals or by using the formula:[10]

$$RCF = 1.118 \times 10^{-5} \times \text{radius in centimeters} \times RPM^2$$

4. A uniform amount of urine, usually 0.5 or 1.0 ml, should remain in the tube after decantation to be used for resuspension of the sediment. Commercial systems supply pipettes for this purpose. They are also used to resuspend the sediment and to transfer a portion to the microscopic slide. If a stain is being used, it should be added before the specimen is agitated for resuspension. Types of stains are discussed later in this chapter.
5. One drop of the resuspended sediment is transferred to a microscope slide and a coverslip is added. Drops should be of uniform size and small enough not to overrun the slide. Commercial systems provide slides containing wells designed to hold a measured amount of specimen. Some laboratories prefer using a hemocytometer and calculating the actual number of elements present in the unspun urine.[13]
6. The manner by which the microscopic examination is performed should be consistent and should include observation of an adequate number of fields under both low and high power. The slide is first examined under low power to detect casts and to ascertain the general composition of the sediment. When objects needing identification are encountered, the setting is changed to high power. Casts have a tendency to locate near the edges of the coverslip; therefore, low-power scanning of the coverslip perimeter or a minimum of 10 fields in that area is recommended. High-power observations should be made of at least 10 and preferably 20 fields.[20] When using bright-field microscopy, care must be taken to reduce the amount of light, since many sediment constituents have a refractive index similar to urine and will not be seen under bright light. Continuous focusing with the fine adjustment will also aid in the detection of these elements.
7. Results are reported as an average of the fields examined. The exact terminology used may vary slightly among laboratories but should be consistent within a single laboratory. Red and white blood cells, epithelial cells, and crystals are reported as the number per high-power field; casts as the number per low-power field; and other elements as 1+, 2+, 3+, and 4+ or, in the corresponding terms, rare, few, many, and packed. The term "too numerous to

TABLE 5-1. Routine Urinalysis Correlations

Microscopic Elements	Physical	Chemical	Exceptions
Casts		+Protein	Number
Red Blood Cells	Turbidity Red Color	+Blood	Number Hemolysis
White Blood Cells	Turbidity	+Protein +Leukocytes +Nitrite	Number Type of Bacteria
Epithelial Cells	Turbidity		Number
Crystals	Turbidity Color	pH	Number and Type
Bacteria	Turbidity	+Nitrite pH	Number and Type

count (TNTC)" may be used when markedly increased amounts of cells and crystals are seen. Casts, epithelial cells, and crystals must also be identified as to their type.

8. Microscopic results should be correlated with the physical and chemical findings to ensure the accuracy of the report. Specimens in which the results do not correlate must be rechecked for both technical and clerical errors. Table 5-1 shows some of the more common correlations in the urinalysis; however, the amount of formed elements or chemicals must also be taken into consideration, as must the possibility of interference with chemical tests and the age of the specimen.

SEDIMENT STAINS

Many factors can influence the appearance of the sediment constituents. Cells are seen in various stages of development and degeneration and can be distorted by the chemical content of the urine; therefore, identification can sometimes be difficult, even for experienced laboratory personnel. The use of supravital stains when examining wet preparations or the staining of preserved slides can often aid in the identification. Staining will also increase the overall visibility of the elements by changing their refractive index. The most frequently used supravital stain is the Sternheimer-Malbin stain, which consists of crystal violet and safranin O.[33] The dye is absorbed well by white blood cells, epithelial cells, and casts, providing a clearer delineation of structure and contrasting the colors of the nucleus and cytoplasm. The expected staining reactions of sediment constituents are shown in Table 5-2. White blood cells that stained light blue instead of violet with Sternheimer-Malbin stain were once thought to be diagnostic of pyelonephritis. These large, pale blue leukocytes are called "glitter cells" because brownian movement of the granules within their cytoplasm produces a sparkling appearance. These glitter cells are seen in most hypotonic urines and are not associated with pyelonephritis or any other specific condition. A more recent supravital stain developed by Sternheimer utilizes a copper-phthalocyanine dye, National Fast Blue, and pyronin B, a xanthene dye. The slowly diffusing National Fast Blue, with an affinity for mucopolysaccharides, and the rapidly diffusing pyronin, which stains polynucleotides, provide more differentiation of structure than the original stain.[34] Although it requires more time and equipment than the routine supravital stains, the preparation of permanent slides by cytocentrifugation and staining them with Papanicolaou's stain provides more standardized sediment concentrations and more uniform staining of cells.[30]

TABLE 5-2. Expected Staining Reactions of Sediment Constituents*

Elements in Urinary Sediment	Usual Distinguishing Color of Stained Elements		Comments
Red Blood Cells	Neutral—pink to purple Acid—pink (unstained) Alkaline—purple		
	Nuclei	*Cytoplasm*	
White Blood Cells—Dark Staining Cells	Purple	Purple granules	
Glitter Cells (Sternheimer-Malbin positive cells)	Colorless or light blue	Pale blue or grey	Some glitter cells exhibit brownian movement.
Renal Tubular Epithelial Cells	Dark shade of blue-purple	Light shade of blue-purple	
Bladder Tubular Epithelial Cells	Blue-purple	Light purple	
Squamous Epithelial Cells	Dark shade of orange-purple	Light purple or blue	
	Inclusions and Matrix		
Hyaline Casts	Pale pink or pale purple		Very uniform color. Slightly darker than mucous threads.
Coarse Granular Inclusion Casts	Dark purple granules in purple matrix		
Finely Granular Inclusion Casts	Fine dark purple granules in pale pink or pale purple matrix		
Waxy Casts	Pale pink or pale purple		Darker than hyaline casts, but of a pale even color. Distinct broken ends.
Fat Inclusion Cast	Fat globules unstained in a pink matrix		Rare. Presence is confirmed if examination under polarized light indicates double refraction.
Red Cell Inclusion Cast	Pink to orange-red		Intact cells can be seen in matrix.
Blood (Hemoglobin) Casts	Orange-red		No intact cells.
Bacteria	Motile: don't stain Nonmotile: stain purple		Motile organisms are not impaired.

TABLE 5-2. *Continued*

Elements in Urinary Sediment	Usual Distinguishing Color of Stained Elements	Comments
Trichomonas vaginalis	Light blue-green	Motility is unimpaired in fresh specimens when recommended volumes of stain are used. Immotile organisms also identifiable.
Mucus	Pale pink or pale blue	
Background	Pale pink or pale purple	

*From *Product Profile: Sedi-Stain,*[27] with permission.

MICROSCOPY

Due to its availability, the bright-field microscope is most frequently used for the examination of the urinary sediment. However, as mentioned earlier, analysis of the unstained sediment presents certain problems with bright-field microscopy because the refractive index of some elements is similar to that of urine and they may be overlooked. To avoid this problem, some laboratories prefer to use the phase-contrast microscope. By retardation of light rays diffused by the object in focus, a halo effect is produced around the element, thereby providing better image reinforcement.[6] Even better differentiation can be obtained by using the interference-contrast microscope. A three-dimensional image showing very fine structural detail is produced by splitting the light ray so that one beam passes through the image and the other serves as a reference. The light interference produced by the object is compared with the reference beam, and a three-dimensional image is visualized.[14] Identification of crystals and lipids is aided by the use of polarized light. Both substances have the ability to rotate the path of the unidirectional polarized light beam to produce characteristic colors from crystals and Maltese cross formations in lipids. An automated system for urine microscopy has recently been marketed. Automated Intelligent Microscopy (International Remote Imaging Systems, Chatsworth, California) features a flow-through system in which urine is sandwiched between a sheath fluid as it reaches the focal plane of the microscope. The microscope fields are recorded by video camera, and then the characteristics of the formed elements are presented to a computer for analysis.

SEDIMENT CONSTITUENTS

The normal urine sediment may contain a variety of formed elements. Even the appearance of small numbers of the usually pathologically significant red blood cells, white blood cells, and casts can be normal. Likewise, many routine urines will contain nothing more than a rare epithelial cell or mucus strand. Students often have difficulty adjusting to this, because in the classroom setting, sediments containing abnormalities and multiple elements are usually stressed. They must learn to trust their observations after looking at the recommended number of fields. Actual normal numerical values are not clearly defined, but are approximately 0 to 2 RBC per hpf, 0 to 5 WBC per hpf, and 0 to 2 hyaline casts per lpf. Even these figures must be taken in context with other factors, such as recent stress or strenuous exercise, menstrual contamination, and the presence of bacteria in combination with white blood cells. To put this in better perspective, the elements, shown in Figure 5-1 and in color plates at the end of the book, will be discussed individually.

Red Blood Cells

White Blood Cells

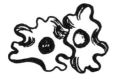

Squamous
Epithelial Cells

Renal Tubular
Epithelial Cells

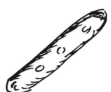

Hyaline Cast

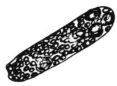

Cellular/Granular Cast

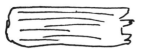

Broad Waxy Cast

Yeast Cells

FIGURE 5-1. Urinary sediment constituents.

RED BLOOD CELLS

Because red blood cells cannot enter the filtrate of an intact nephron, the finding of more than an occasional red blood cell in the urine is considered abnormal. The presence of red blood cells in the urine is associated with damage to the glomerular membrane or vascular injury within the genitourinary tract. The number of cells counted is also an aid in determining the extent of the renal injury. Large amounts of red blood cells are frequently associated with glomerulonephritis, but are also seen in many other conditions, including acute infections, toxic and immunologic reactions, malignancies, and circulatory disorders that disrupt the integrity of the renal capillaries. The observation of microscopic hematuria can be essential to the diagnosis of renal calculi. The possibility of menstrual contamination must also be considered in specimens from female patients.

Red blood cells appear in the urine as colorless disks measuring approximately 7 microns in diameter. Of all the sediment elements, red blood cells cause students the most difficulty in recognition due to their lack of characteristic structures, variations in size, and close resemblance to other urine constituents. In concentrated urine, the cells shrink and often appear crenated; while in dilute alkaline urine, they swell and lyse rapidly, releasing their hemoglobin leaving only the cell membrane. These empty cells are referred to as ghost cells and can be easily missed if specimens are not examined under subdued light. Red blood cells are frequently confused with yeast cells and oil droplets; however, yeast cells will usually exhibit budding, and oil droplets are highly refractile when the fine adjustment is focused up and down. Should the identification continue to be doubtful, addition of acetic acid to a portion of the sediment will lyse the red blood cells, leaving the yeast and oil droplets intact.

As discussed earlier, the presence or absence of red blood cells in the sediment cannot always be correlated with specimen color or a positive chemical test for blood. The presence of hemoglobin that has been filtered by the glomerulus will produce a red urine with a positive chemical test for blood in the absence of microscopic hematuria. Likewise, a specimen appearing macroscopically normal may contain a small but pathologically significant number of red blood cells when examined microscopically.

WHITE BLOOD CELLS

Usually, less than 5 leukocytes per high-power field are found in normal urine; however, higher numbers may be present in female urine.[23] Although leukocytes, like red blood cells, may enter the urine through glomerular or capillary trauma, they are also capable of amoeboid migration through the tissues to sites of infection or inflammation. An increase in urinary white blood cells is called pyuria and indicates the presence of an infection or inflammation in the genitourinary system. Bacterial infections, including pyelonephritis, cystitis, prostatitis, and urethritis, are frequent causes of pyuria. However, pyuria is also present in nonbacterial disorders, such as glomerulonephritis, lupus erythematosus, and tumors. White blood cell clumps and increased bacteria are usually found in specimens that produce positive bacterial cultures.[36]

White blood cells are larger than red blood cells, measuring about 12 microns in diameter. They are much easier to observe and identify because they contain cytoplasmic granules and lobed nuclei. Supravital staining or the addition of acetic acid can be used to enhance the nuclear detail. This can be helpful in distinguishing leukocytes from renal tubular epithelial cells, since observation of the lobulated white blood cell nucleus will differentiate the two cell types. White blood cells lyse rapidly in dilute alkaline urine, and as mentioned earlier, these conditions will also lead to the production of glitter cells.

EPITHELIAL CELLS

It is not unusual to find epithelial cells in the urine, since they are derived from the linings of the genitourinary system. Unless they are present in large numbers or in abnormal forms, they represent normal sloughing of old cells. Three types of epithelial cells are seen in urine, and they are classified as to their site of origin within the genitourinary system.

Squamous cells are the most frequently seen and least significant of the epithelial cells. They are derived from the lining of the vagina and lower portions of the male and female urethras. Increased numbers may be seen in female urine that has not been collected using the midstream clean-catch technique. Squamous cells are large, and they contain abundant, irregular cytoplasm and a central nucleus about the size of a red blood cell. They are often reported in terms of rare, few, many, and packed, instead of actual numbers per high-power field.

Transitional, or caudate, epithelial cells originate from the lining of the renal pelvis, bladder, and upper urethra. They are smaller than squamous cells and are round or pear-shaped with a central nucleus. Like squamous cells, transitional epithelial cells are seldom pathologically important unless large numbers exhibiting unusual morphology are seen. The specimen should then be referred for cytologic examination to determine possible renal carcinoma.

Renal tubular cells are the most significant of the epithelial cells because the finding of increased numbers indicates tubular necrosis and is particularly important in renal graft rejection. Their appearance accompanies conditions causing tubular damage, including pyelonephritis, toxic reactions, viral infections, allograft rejection, and the secondary effects of glomerulonephritis. Renal tubular cells are round and slightly larger than white blood cells. They are distinguished from leukocytes by the presence of a single round nucleus. Staining of sediments using the Sternheimer-Malbin or Papanicolaou method can be helpful if differentiation is difficult.[30] When passage of lipids across the glomerular membrane occurs, as in cases of lipid nephrosis, renal tubular cells absorb lipids and become highly refractile. These lipid-containing renal tubular cells are called oval fat bodies. They are usually seen in conjunction with free-floating fat droplets in the sediment. Examination of the sediment using polarized light will produce characteristic Maltese cross formations in droplets containing cholesterol. Globules that do not contain cholesterol can be identified by adding Sudan III to the sediment and observing the appearance of orange staining globules. Because renal tubular cells and oval fat bodies are pathologically significant, they should be reported in numbers per high-power field. In lipid-storage diseases, large fat-containing cells called histiocytes may also be found in the urine sediment. They can be differentiated from oval fat bodies by their large size.

CASTS

Casts are the only elements found in the urinary sediment that are unique to the kidney. They are formed primarily within the lumen of the distal convoluted tubule and collecting ducts, providing a microscopic view of conditions occurring within the nephron. Several factors influence the formation of casts, including low urine pH, increased solute concentration, increased protein, and decreased rate of urine flow. Their shapes are representative of the tubular lumen, generally consisting of parallel sides and blunt ends; but they may be convoluted, depending on the area of the tubule in which they are formed[31] or the age of the cast.[21] The width of the cast is also determined by the area of formation. Casts formed within the collecting ducts are much broader than those from the tubules and represent an extreme stasis in urine flow. Formation of casts at the junction of the ascending loop of Henle and the distal convoluted tubule may produce structures with a tapering end. These are often referred to as cylindroids, but they have the same significance as casts.[7] The appearance of a cast is also influenced by the materials present in the filtrate at the time of its formation and the length of time it remains in the tubule prior to excretion. Thus, the types of casts found in the sediment will represent different clinical conditions and are summarized in Table 5-3.

The major constituent of casts is Tamm-Horsfall protein, a glycoprotein secreted by the renal tubular cells.[12] It is found in both normal and abnormal urine but is not detected by dipstick methods; therefore, it does not account for the increased urinary protein frequently associated with casts. Scanning electron microscope studies have provided a step-by-step analysis of the formation of the Tamm-Horsfall protein matrix.[21] When conditions conducive to cast formation are present, aggregates of secreted Tamm-Horsfall protein form fibrils that remain attached to the renal tubular cells. As protein secretion and fibril formation continue, the fibrils form a mesh-like network and eventually a solid protein matrix. Elements such as red blood cells, white blood cells, bacteria, and amorphous urates present in the filtrate may be incorporated into the cast. Contrary to popular belief, scanning electron microscopy has shown these elements to be tightly attached to the surface of the protein matrix rather than having been trapped during the formation of the membrane.[15]

HYALINE CASTS

The most frequently seen cast is the hyaline type, which consists almost entirely of Tamm-Horsfall protein. The presence of 0 to 2 hyaline casts per low-power field is considered normal, as is the finding of increased numbers following strenuous exercise, dehydration, and heat exposure.[16] Situations such as these provide ideal conditions for cast formation because the loss of fluid through external sources produces a concen-

TABLE 5-3. Summary of Urine Casts

Type	Origin	Clinical Significance
Hyaline	Tubular secretion of Tamm-Horsfall protein fibrils	Glomerulonephritis Pyelonephritis Chronic renal disease Congestive heart failure Stress and exercise 0–2/lpf normal
Red Blood Cell	Attachment of red blood cells to Tamm-Horsfall protein matrix	Glomerulonephritis Strenuous exercise
White Blood Cell	Attachment of white blood cells to Tamm-Horsfall protein matrix	Pyelonephritis
Epithelial Cell	Tubular cells remaining attached to Tamm-Horsfall protein fibrils	Renal tubular damage
Granular	Disintegration of white cell casts Bacteria Urates Tubular cell lysosomes Protein aggregates	Stasis of urine flow Urinary tract infection Stress and exercise
Waxy	Hyaline casts	Stasis of urine flow
Fatty	Renal tubular cells Oval fat bodies	Nephrotic syndrome
Broad Casts	Formation in collecting ducts	Extreme stasis of urine flow

trated urine and decreased urine flow. Hyaline casts are increased in acute glomerulonephritis, pyelonephritis, chronic renal disease, and congestive heart failure.[7] Hyaline casts appear colorless in unstained sediments and have a refractive index similar to urine; thus, they can easily be overlooked if specimens are not examined under subdued light. Sternheimer-Malbin stain produces a pink color in hyaline casts.

RED BLOOD CELL CASTS

Cellular casts may contain red blood cells, white blood cells, or epithelial cells. The presence of cellular casts is usually indicative of serious renal disease, although red casts have been found in healthy individuals following participation in contact sports.[16] While the finding of red blood cells in the urine indicates bleeding from some area of the genitourinary tract, the presence of red cell casts is much more specific, showing bleeding from within the nephron. Red cell casts are primarily associated with glomerulonephritis; however, any condition that damages the glomerulus, tubules, or renal capillaries may cause the production of red cell casts. Red cell casts are easily recognized because they are refractile and have a color ranging from yellow to brown. They may contain clearly discernible cells or tightly packed cells on the protein matrix. With careful focusing, the cell walls will be visible even in a tightly packed cast. As the cast ages, cell lysis begins and the cast appears more homogenous; however, the released hemoglobin retains the characteristic yellow-brown color. At one time, it was thought that casts containing red blood cells and those containing hemoglobin represented different diseases and that a differentiation between them should be reported. This has not proved true, and both types should be reported as the number of red cell casts per low-power field.[7] Sediments that contain red cell casts should also contain free red blood cells.

WHITE BLOOD CELL CASTS

The appearance of white blood cell casts in the urine signifies infection or inflammation within the nephron. They are most frequently seen in pyelonephritis, but will occur in any condition that causes inflammation of the nephron and will also accompany red cell casts in glomerulonephritis. White blood cell casts are refractile, exhibit granules, and unless disintegration has begun, multilobed nuclei will be visible. Distinguishing white blood cell casts from epithelial casts can present some difficulty, and as mentioned earlier, staining may be necessary to produce visible nuclei. Observation of free white blood cells in the sediment can also aid in the identification. The presence of white blood cell casts indicates a need to perform bacterial cultures.

EPITHELIAL CELL CASTS

As discussed earlier, fibrils of Tamm-Horsfall protein remain attached to the tubular cells; otherwise, they would pass into the urine prior to cast formation. Detachment from the tubular cells may occur at varying points in the formation process. Considering the close adherence of the Tamm-Horsfall protein to the tubular cells, the observation of an occasional epithelial cell attached to a hyaline cast can be expected. However, when tubular damage is present, cells are readily removed from the tubule during cast detachment, and true epithelial cell casts appear in the urine. An entire piece of tubular tissue may be found attached to the cast. Epithelial cell casts are often observed in conjunction with red cell and white cell casts, because both glomerulonephritis and pyelonephritis produce tubular damage. They can be distinguished from white blood cell casts by the presence of a centrally located round nucleus.

GRANULAR CASTS

The appearance of coarsely and finely granular casts in the urinary sediment is generally considered to represent disintegration of the cellular casts remaining in the tubules as a result of urine stasis. Scanning electron microscope studies have confirmed that granular casts seen in conjunction with white blood cell casts contain white cell granules of varying sizes.[22] Bacteria may also be present and can appear as granules under bright-field microscopy. Granular casts unrelated to cellular casts are sometimes seen following periods of stress and strenuous exercise and contain proteins of non-pathologic significance or lysosomes from tubular cells.[15,16]

WAXY CASTS

Previously thought to represent the final disintegration stage of cellular casts, waxy casts may instead be an advanced stage of the hyaline cast. Examination of the surface ultrastructure shows broken plates of surface protein covering a fibril protein matrix.[15,21] Waxy casts are refractile with a rigid texture, and this lack of flexibility may cause them to become fragmented as they pass through the tubules.

FATTY CASTS

Another disintegration product of cellular casts is the fatty cast, which is produced by the breakdown of epithelial cell casts that contain oval fat bodies. As discussed earlier, renal tubular epithelial cells will absorb lipids entering the tubules through the glomerulus. When these lipid-containing cells become attached to a cast, disintegration produces the fatty cast. Fatty casts are highly refractile and contain yellow-brown fat droplets. A more positive identification can be made by staining with Sudan III or by examining the casts under polarized light.

BROAD CASTS

As a mold of the distal convoluted tubules, casts may vary in size as disease distorts the tubular structure. Also, when the flow of urine from the tubules to the collecting ducts becomes severely compromised, conditions become right for casts to form in the collecting ducts. These casts are much larger than other casts and are called broad casts. All types of casts can occur in the broad form, and the finding of many broad waxy casts suggests a serious prognosis. Broad casts are sometimes referred to as renal failure casts. In glomerulonephritis and the nephrotic syndrome, the sediment may contain a wide mixture of the casts and cells just discussed. When this condition is observed, it is termed a telescoped urinary sediment.

BACTERIA

Bacteria are not normally present in the urine. However, unless specimens are collected under sterile conditions, bacterial contamination may occur and is of no clinical significance. Specimens that have remained at room temperature for extended periods of time may also contain noticeable amounts of bacteria that represent nothing more than multiplication of contaminants. Most laboratories report bacteria only when observed in fresh specimens in conjunction with white blood cells.

YEAST

Yeast cells, usually *Candida albicans,* may be seen in urine from patients with diabetes mellitus and women with vaginal moniliasis. They are easily confused with red blood cells and should be observed closely for the presence of budding forms.

PARASITES

The most frequent parasite encountered in the urine is *Trichomonas vaginalis,* a contaminant from vaginal secretions. The organism is a flagellate and is easily identified by its rapid movement in the microscopic field. However, when not moving, *Trichomonas* may resemble a white blood cell. The ova of a true urinary parasite, *Schistosoma haematobium,* will appear in urine; however, it is seldom seen in the United States. Ova from pinworms and other intestinal parasites are occasionally seen in the urine as a result of fecal contamination.

SPERMATOZOA

Spermatozoa are occasionally found in urine following sexual intercourse or nocturnal emissions and are of no clinical significance.

MUCUS

Mucus is a protein material produced by glands and epithelial cells in the genitourinary tract. It is not considered clinically significant, and increased amounts usually occur from vaginal contamination. Mucus appears microscopically as thread-like structures with low refractive indexes requiring observation under subdued light. Care must be taken not to confuse clumps of mucus with hyaline casts. The differentiation can usually be made by observing the irregular appearance of the mucus threads.

CRYSTALS

Crystals are frequently found in the urine. Although they are seldom of any clinical significance, identification must be made to ensure that they do not represent an abnormality. Crystals are formed by the precipitation of urine salts subjected to changes in pH, temperature, or concentration that affect their solubility. The precipitated salts appear in the urine in the form of either true crystals or amorphous material that is also included under the category of urinary crystals.

Normal freshly voided urine may contain crystals formed in the bladder or, less frequently, in the tubules. Increased solute concentration is usually responsible for this in vivo precipitation, which is most often encountered in first morning specimens. The majority of crystal formation takes place in specimens that have been allowed to remain at room temperature or have been refrigerated. Crystals are extremely abundant in refrigerated specimens and often present problems because they obscure other more clinically significant sediment constituents. Some normal crystals will dissolve when the specimen is warmed, but others may require the addition of acid, which will also destroy other formed elements such as red blood cells.

Considerable attention has been given to developing a correlation between the presence of urinary crystals and the formation of renal calculi. The finding of clumps of crystals in freshly voided urine suggests that conditions may be right for calculus formation, and increased crystalluria has been noted in stone formers during the summer months.[17] However, due to the variation in conditions that affect urine within the body and urine in a specimen container and the fact that a true understanding of the actual mechanisms of calculi formation is still not available, little importance is placed on the role of crystals in the diagnosis of renal calculi.[3] Therefore, the primary reason for the identification of urinary crystals is to detect the presence of the relatively few abnormal types that may represent such disorders as liver disease, inborn errors of metabolism, or renal damage caused by crystallization of drug metabolites within the tubules.[4]

The most valuable aid in the identification of crystals is knowledge of the urine pH, since this will determine the type of chemicals precipitated. Crystals are routinely categorized not only as normal or abnormal, but also by their appearance in acidic or alkaline urine. The most commonly seen crystals have very characteristic shapes or colors; however, variations do occur and can present identification problems, particularly when they resemble abnormal crystals. The identification of crystals in specimens with a neutral pH can also cause difficulty because crystals normally classified as acidic or alkaline types may be found in neutral urine. Normal crystals will be discussed in this chapter with respect to their appearance in acidic or alkaline urine. Abnormal crystals, which are only found in acidic or neutral urine, will be covered following normal crystals. The major identifying characteristics of normal crystals are summarized in Table 5-4, and abnormal crystals, in Table 5-5.

NORMAL CRYSTALS

The most common crystals seen in acidic urine are urates, consisting of uric acid, amorphous urates, and sodium urate. Microscopically, all urate crystals appear yellow to red-brown and are the only normal crystals found in acidic urine that appear colored. Uric acid crystals are seen in a variety of shapes, including rhombic plates, rosettes, wedges, and needles. Identification is best made by color rather than shape. Markedly increased levels of uric acid crystals are seen in leukemia, particularly in those patients receiving chemotherapy, and sometimes in cases of gout. As the name implies, amorphous urates consist of yellow-brown granules often occurring in clumps that may be confused with granular casts. When present in large amounts, amorphous urates may give the urine, and particularly the sediment, a macroscopic pink color (see Chapter 3). Calcium oxalate crystals are also frequently found in acidic urine, but they can also be seen in neutral urine, and even rarely in alkaline urine. In their classic form, they are easily recognized as colorless octahedrals that resemble envelopes; however, dumbbell and ring forms may also occur. Calcium oxalate crystals are associated with diets high in oxalic acid and with chemical toxicity and are seen in genetically susceptible persons following large doses of ascorbic acid.[5]

Phosphates represent the majority of the crystals seen in alkaline urine, including triple phosphate, amorphous phosphates, and calcium phosphate. Triple phosphate

TABLE 5-4. Major Characteristics of Normal Urinary Crystals[4]

Crystal	pH	Color	Solubility	Appearance
Uric Acid	Acid	Yellow-Brown	Alkali Soluble	
Amorphous Urates	Acid	Brick Dust or Yellow Brown	Alkali and Heat	
Calcium Oxalate	Acid/Neutral (Alkaline)	Colorless (Envelopes)	Dilute HCl	
Amorphous Phosphates	Alkaline Neutral	White-Colorless	Dilute Acetic Acid	
Calcium Phosphate	Alkaline Neutral	Colorless	Dilute Acetic Acid	
Ammonium Biurate	Alkaline	Yellow-Brown (Thorny Apples)	Heat with Acetic Acid	
Calcium Carbonate	Alkaline	Colorless (Dumbbells)	Gas with Acetic Acid	

TABLE 5-5. Major Characteristics of Abnormal Urinary Crystals[4]

Crystal	pH	Color	Solubility	Appearance
Cystine	Acid	Colorless	Ammonia, Dilute HCl	
Cholesterol	Acid	Colorless (Notched Plates)	Chloroform	
Leucine	Acid/Neutral	Yellow	Hot Alkali or Alcohol	
Tyrosine	Acid/Neutral	Colorless-Yellow	Alkali or Heat	
Sulfonamides	Acid/Neutral	Green	Acetone	
Radiographic Dye	Acid	Colorless	10% NaOH	
Ampicillin	Acid/Neutral	Colorless	Refrigeration Forms Bundles	

crystals are probably the most easily identified urine crystals because in their routine form, they appear as colorless prisms referred to as "coffin lids." They are often seen in large numbers in urine that has been standing at room temperature for several hours. Like amorphous urates, amorphous phosphates are granular in appearance. When present in large amounts, they produce a macroscopic white turbidity in the urine. Calcium phosphate crystals are not frequently encountered and appear as colorless, thin prisms, plates, or needles. When found in neutral urine, they may be confused with abnormal sulfonamide crystals; however, calcium phosphate crystals are soluble in dilute acetic acid, and sulfonamides are not. Other normal crystals associated with alkaline urine are ammonium biurate and calcium carbonate. Like the urate crystals, ammonium biurate crystals have a yellow-brown color. They are frequently described as "thorny apples" due to their appearance as spicule covered spheres. Calcium carbonate crystals are small and colorless, with dumbbell or spherical shapes. They may occur in clumps that resemble amorphous phosphates, but they can be distinguished by the formation of gas after the addition of acetic acid.

ABNORMAL CRYSTALS

The abnormal crystals of primary concern include cystine, cholesterol, leucine, tyrosine, sulfonamides, radiographic dyes, and ampicillin. Hemosiderin, appearing as yellow-brown granules, may also be seen in anemias caused by red blood cell destruction. The granules are sometimes located in casts and epithelial cells but are also free-floating. Staining the sediment with Prussian blue will confirm the presence of hemosiderin.

Most abnormal crystals have characteristic shapes, all are found in acid or neutral urine, and chemical tests are available for positive identification. Cystine crystals that appear as colorless hexagonal plates are found in persons who inherited a metabolic defect that prevents the reabsorption of cystine by the proximal convoluted tubule. Persons with cystinuria have a tendency to form renal calculi. Cholesterol crystals are rarely seen unless specimens have been refrigerated, because the lipids remain in droplet form. However, when observed, they have a most characteristic appearance, resembling a rectangular plate with a notch in one or more corners. Leucine crystals, which appear as yellow-brown sphericals that contain concentric circles with radial striations, and tyrosine crystals, which resemble sheaths of fine needles, are seen rarely in cases of severe liver disease. Until the development of more soluble sulfonamides, the appearance of these crystals in urine was common in patients who were not adequately hydrated. This condition could result in tubular damage if crystals formed in the nephron. Likewise, patients exhibiting radiographic dye and ampicillin crystals may develop problems if sufficient fluid is not taken. Radiographic dye crystals may resemble uric acid but can be suspected in specimens that have an abnormally high specific gravity. As discussed earlier, the use of polarized light can also aid in crystal identification and is particularly valuable for distinguishing nonpolarized cystine crystals from uric acid crystals. The problems associated with the identification of abnormal crystals can often be solved by a check on the medications and treatments the patient is receiving. When this is not done, considerable time and energy can be wasted trying to identify the crystals solely by appearance.

ARTIFACTS

Contaminants of all types can be found in urine, particularly in those specimens collected under improper conditions or in dirty containers. Most confusing to students are oil droplets and starch granules (talcum powder), since they resemble red blood cells. However, they are much more refractile, and if polarized light is used, starch granules will exhibit Maltese cross formation. Hair and other fibers may initially be mistaken for casts, but close examination should rule this out.

QUALITY CONTROL IN URINALYSIS

During the discussion of the routine urinalysis in this and the previous two chapters, the methods of ensuring accurate test results were covered on an individual basis for each of the tests. Since quality control in the urinalysis laboratory, or any other laboratory department, is an integration of many factors, this section will provide an overall view of the procedures essential for providing quality urinalysis. Table 5-6 provides a daily, weekly, and monthly description of routine quality control procedures in the urinalysis laboratory.

TABLE 5-6. The Mount Vernon Hospital Chemistry Lab—Urinalysis Quality Control*

I. Perform the following DAILY.

   1. Clean the work area with disinfectant.

   2. Refractometer: read specific gravity of water—1.000
                             read specific gravity of 5% NaCl—should read 1.022 ± .001

   3. Harleco URINTROL (may be stored at room temperature after opening)—mix thoroughly by gently inverting 10–15 times):
      a. Specific gravity—Refractometer
      b. Chemstrip 7
      c. Sulfosalicylic acid
      d. Clinitest

   4. All results are recorded on the Quality Control Forms, and initialed.

   5. When a test is out of control:
      a. DO NOT REPORT OUT RESULTS
      b. Check reagents for contamination, outdating, and/or correct lot numbers
      c. Repeat using new Urintrol and fresh reagents
      d. Notify supervisor

   6. Daily in-house control:

      Each day, the morning shift will choose one urine specimen of sufficient quantity for the in-house control for that day. Each of the following two shifts will also do a complete urinalysis (including microscopic) on this same specimen. Store in the refrigerator when not in use. Allow specimen to come to room temperature before use.

      Record results on the In-House Control Forms in the notebook for the appropriate shift.

II. Perform the following AS REQUIRED. Do only when (a) a patient test is required and (b) it has not been done that day.

   1. Harleco Urintrol:
      a. Acetest
      b. Ictotest
      c. Chemstrip GK

   2. Record all results on the Quality Control Form, and initial.

III. Perform the following WEEKLY.

   1. Clean and check sulfosalicylic acid dispenser:

      Volumetrically pipette 1.0 ml sulfosalicylic acid into a 10-ml volumetric flask. Make sure the Oxford Pipettor is primed, and dispense three 3.0-ml aliquots into the volumetric flask. This should equal 10.0 ml. If not, adjust the pipettor accordingly and recheck.

      Log under Miscellaneous Quality Control, and initial.

TABLE 5-6. *Continued*

    2. Read the pH on the Chemstrip 7 after dipping the strip in the pH 7 buffer (pH meter buffer).

    This should read 6.5–7.5. Record under Miscellaneous on Quality Control Forms, and initial.

    3. Check pH of distilled water using pH meter. Record and initial sheet on the wall in the dishwashing room and by the chemistry spigot. Also check the resistance of both water supplies and record.

    4. Clean the centrifuge with disinfectant.

IV. Perform the following MONTHLY.

    1. Make certain that Microbiology has cultured both water supplies and that the bacterial count is below 100 organisms/ml for each.

*From Clare Bowman, MT (ASCP), Mount Vernon Hospital Department of Pathology,[24] with permission.

Total quality control has been categorized in many ways. Table 5-7 shows a comparison between the original industrial quality control measurements and laboratory quality control. Plaut and Silberman[26] outline the system in the following manner:

1. Sample collection and identification
2. Methodology
    Instrumentation
    Reagents
    Calibration
3. Instrument maintenance
    Manufacturer's recommendations
    Laboratory preventive maintenance
4. Quality Control
    Material
    Data handling

TABLE 5-7. Comparison between Original Industrial Quality Control Measurements and Laboratory Quality Control*

	In Industry	*Medical Laboratory*
Phase I.	New design control	Selection of the proper tests and the proper method for a particular patient problem
Phase II.	Incoming material control	Standards, control sera, and evaluation of reagent kits and instruments, and so forth
Phase III.	Process control	Internal quality control and external quality control (proficiency testing)
Phase IV.	Product output control	Format of presentation of results to physicians to solve a patient problem
Phase V.	Product reliability	Reliability of the interpretation of the result by the physician
Phase VI.	Special process studies	An inspection and accreditation program

*From Eilers,[11] p. 1364, with permission.

To each of these outlines should also be added training and continuing education of the personnel performing the tests.

Documentation of quality control procedures is essential for laboratory accreditation by either the Joint Commission of Accreditation of Hospitals (JCAH) or the College of American Pathologists (CAP) and for Medicare approval. Guidelines published by CAP provide very complete instructions for documentation and are used as a reference for the ensuing discussion of the specific areas of urinalysis quality control.[8]

SPECIMEN COLLECTION, HANDLING, AND IDENTIFICATION

Written instructions should be available to patients for the collection of clean-catch and timed specimens. As discussed in Chapter 1, specimens should be examined fresh. If this is not possible, instructions for the preservation of specimens for both routine and special tests must be available. When specimens are incorrectly labeled, the personnel responsible for collection are notified, and a new sample is requested.

METHODOLOGY

A procedure manual containing all of the procedures performed in the urinalysis section must be available for reference in the working area. The following information is included for each procedure: specimen handling, test principles, preparation of reagents, controls and standards, methodology, calculations, tolerance limits for controls, normal values, special requirements, and references. Evaluation of new procedures and adoption of new methodologies is an ongoing process in the clinical laboratory. All changes in the procedure manual are initialed by the section supervisor, and the manual must be reviewed annually by the laboratory director (notice initials in Table 5-8).

REAGENTS

All reagents and dipsticks must be properly labeled with the date of preparation or opening, purchase date, and expiration date. Dipsticks should be checked against a known control solution on each shift and whenever a new bottle is opened. Reagents are checked daily or when tests requiring their use are requested. Results of all reagent checks are recorded.

Many commercial control materials are available for monitoring reagent and dipstick reactivity; however, most do not include sediment constituents for monitoring the microscopic analysis. Controls for nitrite and leukocytes can be prepared by making aliquots of positive patient specimens and storing them in the refrigerator for 1 week.

In-house controls, as described in Table 5-6, provide an inexpensive way to monitor performance. Preparation of controls containing sediment constituents can be done using a method described by Hoeltge and Ersts.[18] Elements to be preserved are washed in cold 0.85 percent saline and fixed overnight in a 10 percent formol-saline solution (0.85 g NaCl plus 10 ml aqueous formalin, q.s. to 100 ml with distilled water). Aliquots added to chemical controls can then be frozen. The majority of the sediment constituents seen in the photographs at the end of this book were preserved in this manner and stored under refrigeration up to 6 months. External quality control programs such as that offered by the CAP provide an additional means for monitoring laboratory quality. Laboratories subscribing to this program receive lyophilized specimens for routine urinalysis and transparencies for sediment constituent identification every 3 months. The results are returned to the CAP, where they are statistically analyzed with those from all participating laboratories, and a report is returned to the laboratory director.

Corrective action, including the use of new reagents or dipsticks and controls and the verification of lot numbers and expiration dates, must be taken when control values are outside of the tolerance limits. All corrective actions taken are documented.

TABLE 5-8. The Mount Vernon Hospital Routine Urinalysis— Standardization of Report*

1. Color

   Yellow, dark yellow, bright yellow, or other colors (due to medication)

2. Appearance

   Clear, slightly hazy, hazy, cloudy, turbid

3. Reaction to Chemstrip 7 and other chemical tests

   a. Protein—neg, trace, 1+, 2+, 3+, 4+ (back-up test: Sulfa Sal)
   *b. Glucose—neg, trace, 1+, 2+, 3+, 4+ (back-up test: Clinitest)
   CB c. Ketones—trace, 1+, 2+, 3+ (back-up test: Acetest)
   5-20-82 CB d. Bilirubin—trace, 1+, 2+, 3+ (back-up test: Ictotest)
   e. Occult blood—neg, trace, 1+, 2+, 3+
   f. Urobilinogen—neg or Ehrlich units

   *Also check urine of all patients under 2 years old for reducing substances—using Clinitest tablets.

   *A back-up test, when available, is performed on all positive or questionable Chemstrip 7 tests. The result of the dipstick test, if confirmed, is the one reported out, and the back-up test(s) performed are recorded on the log-in sheet.

4. Microscopic examination

   a. Leukocytes—record average number/high-power field
   b. Erythrocytes—record average number/high-power field
   c. Epithelial cells

      Rare: 1 in every five fields/hpf
      Occ.: 1 in every field/hpf
      Few: 2–5 in every field/hpf
      Mod.: 5–10 in every field/hpf
      Many: 10 or more in every field/hpf

   d. Mucous Threads—light, moderate, heavy
   e. Crystals—report same as for epithelial cells (note—amorphous according to pH)
   f. Casts—identify type, i.e., granular, hyaline, WBC, RBC, and so forth. Report number present/low-power field
   g. Cylindroids—distinguish whether mucous or hyaline cast and report accordingly
   h. Bacteria—report as negative, light, moderate, heavy

   Centrifuge 10 ml urine for 5 minutes at 400 G (1500 RPM) (set at 3.5 on Sorvall)

*From Clare Bowman, MT (ASCP), Mount Vernon Hospital Department of Pathology,[24] with permission.

INSTRUMENTATION AND EQUIPMENT

The most frequently encountered instruments in the urinalysis laboratory are those used to measure urine solute. They include urinometers, refractometers, and osmometers. Both urinometers and refractometers are calibrated daily against distilled water (1.000) and a known control, such as 5 percent saline (1.022 ±0.001). Both high and low controls are available for the osmometer. All control values are recorded.

Automated urinalysis systems and dipstick readers are calibrated using negative and positive controls.

Equipment found in the urinalysis laboratory includes, primarily, refrigerators, centrifuges, microscopes, and water baths. Temperatures of refrigerators and water baths should be taken daily and recorded. Calibration of centrifuges is customarily performed every 3 months, and the appropriate RPM for each setting is recorded. A routine maintenance schedule for each piece of equipment should be prepared, and records should be kept of all routine and nonroutine maintenance performed.

REPORTING OF RESULTS

Forms for reporting results should provide adequate space for writing and should present the information in a logical sequence. Standardized reporting methods will minimize physician confusion in interpreting results (see Table 5-8). Review of the report slips by the section supervisor on a periodic basis throughout the shift will aid in detecting errors and will provide for their timely correction. Written procedures should be available for detection of errors, correction of errors, and for reporting of critical values (Tables 5-9 and 5-10).

TABLE 5-9. Reporting Results/Reviewing Results/Correction of Errors*

1. Early AM urinalysis results on ICU and CCU should be completed and telephoned to the respective units by 10 AM.

2. STAT urinalysis should be completed and called within 30 minutes of collection.

3. On preoperative urinalysis, notify the patient's physician or charge nurse of abnormal results as soon as possible so that another specimen can be obtained and tested prior to surgery. This is particularly important for outpatients scheduled for surgery.

4. At least once each shift, the hematology supervisor or charge technician will review all urinalysis reports for clarity.

5. If an error in reporting has been made or results are questioned, the test will be repeated on the same sample, if available. If the specimen is no longer available and repeat testing is indicated, ask for another specimen and retest.

6. Correction of errors—If an incorrect result has been posted to the patient's chart, do not remove the report. Mark an X through the erroneous result and post the corrected result, so labeled, on a new reporting form to the patient's chart near the invalid result. This should be handled by the supervisor or charge technician.

*From Patricia Stirk, MT (ASCP), Commonwealth Hospital Department of Pathology,[9] with permission.

TABLE 5-10. Urinalysis Panic Values—
Notification of Doctor or Charge Nurse*

Notify the doctor or charge nurse if any of the following occur:

Positive glucose and/or Clinitest 2% or higher
Positive bilirubin/Ictotest
Many granular casts, WBC or RBC casts, or waxy casts
Positive protein/SSA greater than 3+ to 4+ range
Unusual crystals such as cystine

*From Patricia Stirk, MT (ASCP), Commonwealth Hospital Department of Pathology,[9] with permission.

PERSONNEL

Quality control is only as good as the person performing it. Personnel must understand its importance and demonstrate professionalism in their performance of all functions within the laboratory. Qualified personnel, adequate staffing, competent management, and continuing education are all essential to quality work.

REFERENCES

1. ADDIS, T: *The number of formed elements in the urinary sediment of normal individuals.* J Clin Invest 2(5):409–415, 1926.
2. BERHAM, L AND O'KELL, RT: *Urinalysis: Minimizing microscopy.* Clin Chem 28(7):1722, 1982.
3. BOYCE, WH: *Calculous Disease: Guest Editorial.* J Urol 127(5):859, 1982.
4. BRADLEY, M AND SCHUMANN, GB: *Examination of the urine.* In HENRY, JB (ED): *Clinical Diagnosis and Management by Laboratory Methods.* WB Saunders, Philadelphia, 1984.
5. BRADLEY, M: *Urine crystals: Identification and significance.* Laboratory Medicine 13(6):348–353, 1982.
6. BRODY, L, WEBSTER, MC, AND KARK, RM: *Identification of elements in the urinary sediment with phase-contrast microscopy.* JAMA 206(8):1777–1781, 1968.
7. CANNON, DC: *The identification and pathogenesis of urine casts.* Laboratory Medicine 10(1):8–11, 1979.
8. COLLEGE OF AMERICAN PATHOLOGISTS: *Commission of Inspection and Accreditation Inspection Checklist, Section IIIA Urinalysis.* College of American Pathologists, Skokie, Illinois, 1984.
9. COMMONWEALTH DOCTORS HOSPITAL: *Department of Pathology Quality Control Procedure.* Fairfax, Virginia, 1984.
10. DUDAS, H: *Quality in urinalysis.* Laboratory Medicine 12(12):765–767, 1981.
11. EILERS, RJ: *Total quality control for the medical laboratory.* South Med J 62(11):1362–1365, 1969.
12. FLETCHER, AP, NEUBERGER, A, AND RATCLIFFE, WA: *Tamm-Horsfall urinary glycoprotein: The chemical composition.* Biochemistry Journal 120:417–424, 1970.
13. GYORY, AZ, KESSON, AM, AND TALBOT, JM: *Microscopy of urine: Now you see it, now you don't.* Am Heart J 99(4):537–538, 1980.
14. HABER, MH: *Interference contrast microscopy for identification of urinary sediments.* Am J Clin Pathol 57:316–319, 1972.
15. HABER, MH AND LINDER, LE: *The surface ultrastructure of urinary casts.* Am J Clin Pathol 68(5):547–552, 1977.
16. HABER, MH, LINDER, LE, AND CIOFALO, LN: *Urinary casts after stress.* Laboratory Medicine 10(6):351–355, 1979.
17. HALLSON, PC AND ROSE, GA: *Seasonal variations in urinary crystals.* Br J Urol 49(4):277–284, 1977.
18. HOELTGE, GA AND ERSTS, BS: *A quality-control system for the general urinalysis laboratory.* Am J Clin Pathol 73(3):403–408, 1980.
19. KARK, RM, ET AL: *A Primer of Urinalysis.* Harper & Row, New York, 1963.
20. ICL SCIENTIFIC: *Kova System for Standardized Urinalysis.* Fountain Valley, California, 1981.
21. LINDNER, LE AND HABER, MH: *Hyaline casts in the urine: Mechanism of formation and morphological transformations.* Am J Clin Pathol 80(3):347–352, 1983.
22. LINDNER, LE, VACCA, D, AND HABER, MH: *Identification and composition of types of granular urinary casts.* Am J Clin Pathol 80(3):353–358, 1983.
23. MCGUCHEN, M, COHEN, L, AND MACGREGOR, RR: *Significance of pyuria in urinary sediment.* J Urol 120:452–456, 1978.
24. MOUNT VERNON HOSPITAL: *Department of Pathology Quality Control Procedure.* Alexandria, Virginia, 1984.

25. MYNAHAN, C: *Evaluation of macroscopic urinalysis as a screening procedure.* Laboratory Medicine 15(3):176–179, 1984.
26. PLAUT, D AND SILBERMAN, J: *Quality control in the automated laboratory.* Am J Med Technol 49(4):213–218, 1983.
27. *Product Profile: Sedi-Stain.* Clay Adams, Division of Becton, Dickinson and Company, Parsippany, New Jersey, 1974.
28. SCHREINER, GE AND WELT, LG: *Diseases of the Kidney.* Little, Brown & Co, Boston, 1963.
29. SCHUMANN, GB AND GREENBERG, NF: *Usefulness of macroscopic urinalysis as a screening procedure.* Am J Clin Pathol 71(6):452–454, 1979.
30. SCHUMANN, GB AND HENRY, JB: *An improved technique for the evaluation of urine sediment.* Laboratory Management 15:18–24, 1977.
31. SCHUMANN, GB, HENRY, JB, AND HARRIS, S: *An improved technique for examining urinary casts and a review of their significance.* Am J Clin Pathol 69:18–23, 1978.
32. SMALLEY, DL AND BRYAN, JA: *Comparative evaluation of biochemical and microscopic urinalysis.* Am J Med Technol 49(4):237–239, 1983.
33. STERNHEIMER, R AND MALBIN, R: *Clinical recognition of pyelonephritis with a new stain for urinary sediments.* Am J Med 11:312–313, 1951.
34. STERNHEIMER, R: *A supravital cytodiagnostic stain for urinary sediments.* JAMA 231:826–828, 1975.
35. SZWED, JJ AND SCHAUST, C: *The importance of microscopic examination of the urinary sediment.* Am J Med Technol 48(2):141–143, 1982.
36. YU, HD: *Evaluation of microscopic examination of bacteruria.* Chinese Journal of Microbiology 11(1):16–20, 1978.

STUDY QUESTIONS (Choose one best answer)

1. Correct performance of a urinary sediment examination should include:

     1. centrifugation of 10 ml of urine for 5 minutes
     2. addition of preservative prior to centrifugation
     3. resuspending the sediment in 0.5 ml of urine
     4. examining under low and high power
     5. reporting all constituents as number per high-power field

   a. 1, 2, and 3
   b. 2, 4, and 5
   c. 1, 3, and 4
   d. 1, 3, and 5

2. The predecessor of the standardized urine microscopic was the:

   a. Sternheimer count
   b. Addis count
   c. Kova system
   d. T-system

3. Leukocytes that stain pale blue with Sternheimer-Malbin stain and exhibit brownian movement are:

   a. indicative of pyelonephritis
   b. Sternheimer cells
   c. mononuclear leukocytes
   d. glitter cells

4. For better detection of hyaline casts, bright-field microscopy can be replaced by:

   a. phase-contrast microscopy
   b. polarized light
   c. compensated polarized light
   d. dark-field microscopy

5. Identification of oval fat bodies can be made using:

   a. bright-field microscopy
   b. phase contrast
   c. polarized light
   d. interference-contrast microscopy

6. In order to observe elements with a low refractive index when using bright-field microscopy, the:

   a. condenser is raised to increase light
   b. condenser is lowered to increase light
   c. condenser is raised to reduce light
   d. condenser is lowered to reduce light

7. Relative centrifugal force (RCF) is determined by which two factors:

   a. radius of rotor head and RPM
   b. radius of rotor head and time of centrifugation
   c. diameter of rotor head and RPM
   d. RPM and time of centrifugation

8. Which of the following elements would most likely be found in an acidic concentrated urine that contains protein:

   a. ghost red blood cells
   b. casts
   c. oval fat bodies
   d. triple phosphate crystals

9. Urinary sediment examination of a specimen from a patient suspected of having renal calculi should contain:

   a. white blood cells
   b. casts
   c. red blood cells
   d. triple phosphate crystals

10. Differentiation among red blood cells, yeast, and oil droplets may be accomplished by all of the following except:

   a. observation of budding in yeast cells
   b. increased refractibility of oil droplets
   c. lysis of yeast cells by acetic acid
   d. lysis of red blood cells by acetic acid

11. A positive chemical test for blood with no red blood cells found in the sediment:

    a. should have both tests repeated if the specimen is clear and red
    b. indicates the presence of hemoglobin or myoglobin
    c. indicates possible acute glomerulonephritis
    d. is not possible

12. Ghost red blood cells are seen in:

    a. dilute acidic urine
    b. dilute alkaline urine
    c. concentrated acidic urine
    d. concentrated alkaline urine

13. An increase in urinary white blood cells is called:

    a. pyelonephritis
    b. cystitis
    c. urethritis
    d. pyuria

14. Oval fat bodies are:

    a. squamous epithelial cells that contain lipids
    b. renal tubular epithelial cells that contain lipids
    c. free-floating fat droplets
    d. white blood cells with phagocytized lipids

15. Damage to the glomerular membrane can be suspected when the sediment contains:

    a. hyaline casts
    b. red blood cell casts
    c. waxy casts
    d. white blood cell casts

16. Casts will appear in the sediment in the following sequence:

    a. hyaline, finely granular, broad
    b. coarsely granular, finely granular, fatty
    c. cellular, granular, fatty
    d. cellular, granular, waxy

17. Broad casts are:

    a. formed by the disintegration of waxy and fatty casts
    b. formed in the distal convoluted tubules instead of the proximal convoluted tubules
    c. formed at the juncture of the ascending loop of Henle and the distal convoluted tubule
    d. formed in the collecting ducts

18. A urine specimen refrigerated overnight is cloudy and has a pH of 8. The turbidity is probably due to:

    a. amorphous phosphates
    b. amorphous urates
    c. triple phosphate crystals
    d. calcium oxalate crystals

19. To confirm the above identification, you could:

    a. warm the specimen
    b. add sodium hydroxide
    c. add dilute hydrochloric acid
    d. add dilute acetic acid

20. Normal crystals found in acidic urine include:

    a. calcium oxalate, uric acid, amorphous urates
    b. calcium oxalate, uric acid, sulfonamides
    c. uric acid, amorphous urates, calcium carbonate
    d. uric acid, calcium carbonate, ammonium biurate

21. Name a crystal that matches the following descriptions:

    a. "coffin-lid"   _____
    b. "thorny apple"   _____
    c. "envelope"   _____
    d. "dumbbell"   _____

22. Match the following crystals:

    ____ cholesterol   a. spherical, with concentric circles with radial striations
    ____ leucine   b. sheaths of fine needles
    ____ cystine   c. Maltese cross
    ____ tyrosine   d. notched corners
                         e. hexagonal plates

23. The following results were obtained on a urine specimen from a 30-year-old female:

Color: brown	Ketone: negative
Appearance: cloudy	Bilirubin: negative
Sp. Gr.: 1.027	Urobilinogen: 0.1 EU
pH: 5.5	Blood: moderate
Protein: 1+	Nitrite: positive
Glucose: negative	

    Indicate if these results suggest that any of the following may be seen in the sediment and support your answer:
    a. RBCs
    b. WBCs
    c. casts
    d. bacteria

24. A 22-year-old female college student comes to the university health center complaining of a burning sensation while voiding. The urinalysis shows:

Color: straw   Ketone: negative
Appearance: hazy   Bilirubin: negative
Sp. Gr.: 1.008   Urobilinogen: 0.1 EU
pH: 8.0   Blood: trace
Protein: trace   Nitrite: positive
Glucose: negative

Indicate if these results suggest that any of the following may be seen in the sediment and support your answer:
a. RBCs
b. WBCs
c. casts
d. bacteria

25. A medical technology student performs a urinalysis on himself after completing a marathon run. The results are:

Color: dark yellow   Blood: small
Appearance: clear   Nitrite: negative
Sp. Gr.: 1.030   Leukocyte esterase: negative
pH: 5.5   0–4 hyaline casts/lpf
Protein: 2+   0–5 WBC/hpf
Glucose: negative   rare RBCs
Ketone: negative   rare RBC and granular casts
Bilirubin: negative
Urobilinogen: 1.0 EU

The student is upset with these results, but his instructor is not.
a. Which opinion would you support?
b. How could you prove your opinion?
c. Explain the significance of each abnormal result.

26. As supervisor of the urinalysis laboratory, you are reviewing reports sent out by a new employee, and several results concern you. Tell what questions you would ask the person in each of the following cases.

a. pH 7.0 with uric acid crystals
b. 4+ glucose on a preoperative patient
c. specific gravity 1.040
d. yellow, hazy, negative blood, and many RBCs

6
SPECIAL URINALYSIS SCREENING TESTS

INSTRUCTIONAL OBJECTIVES

Upon completion of this chapter, readers will be able to:

1. explain the abnormal accumulation of metabolites in the urine in terms of overflow and renal disorders

2. name the metabolic defect in phenylketonuria and describe the clinical manifestations it produces

3. discuss the performance of the Guthrie and ferric chloride tests and their roles in the detection and management of phenylketonuria

4. list two tests used to screen for urinary tyrosine and its metabolites

5. name the abnormal urinary substance present in alkaptonuria and tell how its presence may be suspected

6. describe the appearance of urine containing excess melanin and two screening tests to detect its presence

7. describe a basic laboratory observation that has relevance in maple syrup urine disease

8. differentiate between the presence of urinary indican due to intestinal disorders and Hartnup disease

9. state the significance of increased urinary 5-HIAA

10. discuss the instructions that must be given to patients prior to the collection of samples to be tested for 5-HIAA

11. differentiate between cystinuria and cystinosis, including the differences that will be found during analysis of the urine

12. name the chemical screening test for cystine

13. explain the chemical screening test used to distinguish between cystine and homocystine

14. describe the basic pathway for the production of heme and tell the two stages affected by lead poisoning

15. describe the appearance of urine that contains increased porphyrins

16. name the porphyrins measured by the Ehrlich reaction and those detected by fluorescence under a Wood's lamp

17. **define mucopolysaccharides and name three syndromes in which they are involved**

18. **list three screening tests for the detection of urinary mucopolysaccharides**

19. **explain the reason for performing tests for urinary reducing substances on all newborns**

In the previous five chapters, we have discussed the role of urinalysis in providing initial diagnostic information concerning metabolic dysfunctions of both renal and nonrenal origin. Much of this information came from the results of the routine urinalysis performed in the urinalysis laboratory, and some came from the measurement of renal function, which is shared between the urinalysis, clinical chemistry, and nuclear medicine laboratories. Although urine, as an end product of body metabolism, contains most substances or their degradation products that are found in the body, the procedures for analysis of these compounds often require sophisticated methodology and equipment not found in the urinalysis laboratory. Therefore, the role of the urinalysis laboratory becomes one of performing screening tests, the qualitative results of which are then utilized by the physician to determine if additional tests are to be performed. Examples of this include the detection by routine urinalysis of conditions such as diabetes mellitus, liver disorders, glomerular or tubular damage, and urinary tract infection. Additional testing of not only urine but also blood, other body fluids, or tissue may then be necessary. The scope of this book is not to cover these additional procedures performed in other sections of the laboratory, but rather to provide students with a thorough understanding of the tests performed within the urinalysis laboratory and their significance as a part of the total diagnostic evaluation.

Although urinalysis laboratories vary as to the extent to which they are equipped to perform specialized procedures, certain tests, again primarily of a qualitative nature, are considered the responsibility of the urinalysis laboratory. As shown in Table 6-1, the necessity of performing additional tests may be detected by the observations of alert laboratory personnel during the performance of the routine analysis and, in some cases, from observations by patients of abnormal specimen color and odor. In other instances, clinical symptoms and family histories are the deciding factors, and many laboratories perform a standardized battery of metabolic screening tests on all newborns.[2]

OVERFLOW VERSUS RENAL DISORDERS

The accumulation of abnormal metabolic substances in the urine may be due to a variety of causes; however, these can generally be grouped into two categories, termed the overflow type and the renal type. Overflow disorders are due to increased production of metabolites resulting from the disruption of a normal metabolic pathway, causing increased serum concentrations of substances that either override the reabsorption ability of the renal tubules or are not normally reabsorbed from the filtrate.[10] Abnormal

TABLE 6-1. Abnormal Metabolic Constituents or Conditions Detected in the Routine Urinalysis

Color	Odor	Crystals
Homogentisic Acid	Phenylketonuria	Cystine
Melanin	Maple Syrup Urine Disease	Leucine
Indican		Tyrosine
Porphyrins		

TABLE 6-2. Major Disorders of Protein and Carbohydrate Metabolism Associated with Abnormal Urinary Constituents Classified as to Functional Defect

Overflow		Renal
Inherited	Metabolic	
Phenylketonuria	Tyrosinemia	Cystinuria
Tyrosinemia	Melanuria	Cystinosis
Alkaptonuria	Indican	Fanconi's Syndrome
Maple Syrup Urine Disease	5-Hydroxyindoleacetic Acid	
Porphyria	Porphyria	
Mucopolysaccharidoses		
Melituria (Galactosuria)		

accumulations of the renal type are due to malfunctions in the tubular reabsorption mechanism. The most frequently encountered abnormalities are associated with metabolic disturbances that produce urinary overflow of substances involved in protein and carbohydrate metabolism. This is understandable when one considers the vast number of enzymes utilized in the metabolic pathways of proteins and carbohydrates and the fact that their function is essential to complete metabolism. Disruption of enzyme function can be caused by failure to inherit the gene to produce a particular enzyme, referred to as an "inborn error of metabolism,"[14] or by organ malfunction due to disease or toxic reactions. Table 6-2 summarizes the most frequently encountered abnormal urinary metabolites and classifies their appearance as to functional defect. Notice that in some cases, there may be more than one cause for the defect. This table also includes those substances and conditions that are covered in this chapter. Many other metabolic disorders with urinary manifestations also exist and are discussed thoroughly by Thomas and Howell.[41]

AMINO ACID DISORDERS
PHENYLALANINE-TYROSINE METABOLISM

Many of the most frequently requested special urinalysis procedures are associated with the phenylalanine-tyrosine metabolic pathway. Major inherited disorders include phenylketonuria, tyrosyluria, alkaptonuria, and metabolic defects producing excessive amounts of melanin. The relationship of these varied disorders is illustrated in Figure 6-1.

PHENYLKETONURIA

The most well-known of the aminoacidurias, phenylketonuria is estimated to occur in 1 of every 10,000 to 20,000 births and, if undetected, results in severe mental retardation. It was first identified in Norway by Ivan Folling in 1934, when a mother with other mentally retarded children reported a peculiar mousy odor to her child's urine.[33] Analysis of the urine showed increased amounts of the keto acids, including phenylpyruvate. As shown in Figure 6-1, this will occur when the normal conversion of phenylalanine to tyrosine is disrupted. Interruption of the pathway also produces children with fair complexions even in dark-skinned families, due to the decreased production of tyrosine and its pigmentation metabolite, melanin. Phenylketonuria (PKU) is caused by the failure to inherit the gene to produce the enzyme phenylalanine hydroxylase, inherited as an autosomal recessive with no noticeable characteristics or defects exhibited by heterozygous carriers. Fortunately, screening tests are available to detect the abnormality,

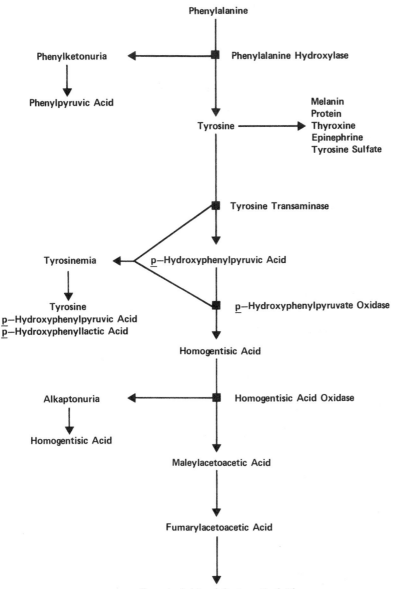

FIGURE 6-1. Phenylalanine and tyrosine metabolism. (Adapted from Frimpton,[13] and Kretchmer and Etzwiler.[24])

and most states have laws that require the screening of all newborns. Once discovered, dietary changes that eliminate phenylalanine, a major constituent of milk, from the infant's diet can prevent the excessive buildup of serum phenylalanine and can thereby avoid damage to the mental capabilities. As the child matures, alternate pathways of phenylalanine metabolism develop, and dietary restrictions can be lifted.

The initial screening for PKU does not come under the auspices of the urinalysis laboratory, since increased blood levels of phenylalanine must, of course, occur prior to the urinary excretion of phenylpyruvic acid, which may take from 2 to 6 weeks. Blood samples are usually obtained before the newborn is discharged from the hospital. To prevent false-negative results, care must be taken to ensure that there has been adequate ingestion of phenylalanine prior to collection of the sample. Therefore, tests should be repeated during an early visit to the pediatrician. More girls than boys escape detection of PKU during early tests because of slower rises in blood phenylalanine levels.[13] Urine testing can be used as a follow-up procedure in questionable diagnostic

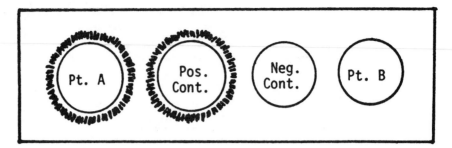

FIGURE 6-2. Guthrie's test.

cases, as a screening test to ensure proper dietary control in previously diagnosed cases, and more recently, as a means of monitoring the dietary intake of pregnant women known to lack phenylalanine hydroxylase.[33]

Several methods are available for measuring serum levels of phenylalanine, including an automated technique that measures the fluorescence of phenylalanine when it is heated in the presence of Ninhydrin and L-leucyl-L-alanine or glycyl-L-leucine.[21] However, the most well-known method is the bacterial inhibition test developed by Guthrie.[15] In this procedure, blood from a heelstick is absorbed into filter paper circles. The blood-impregnated disks are then placed on culture media streaked with the organism *Bacillus subtilis.* If increased levels of phenylalanine are present in the blood, they will counteract the action of an inhibitor of *Bacillus subtilis* that is present in the media, and growth will be observed around the paper disks. Notice that in Figure 6-2, the bacterial growth around the disk from Patient A corresponds to the positive control, indicating an increased blood level of phenylalanine.

Urine tests for phenylpyruvic acid are based on the ferric chloride reaction performed either by tube or dipstick (Phenistix, Ames Company, Elkhart, Indiana). As will be seen in other discussions in this chapter, the ferric chloride test is a nonspecific reaction and will react with many other amino acids and commonly ingested medications (Table 6-3). This is particularly true when the tube test is used, since more substances produce positive, although sometimes transient, reactions. Some brands of disposable diapers also produce false-positive reactions for PKU when tested with ferric chloride.[22] More consistent results are obtained using Phenistix, since the testing area contains a buffer to maintain an acid pH and magnesium ions to reduce the interference produced by urinary phosphates.[41] Phenistix produces a permanent blue-gray to green-gray color when a positive sample is tested. Comparison of results between ferric chloride tube tests and the Phenistix test can sometimes provide useful information in the screening for metabolic disorders.[23]

TYROSYLURIA

The accumulation of excess tyrosine in the serum producing urinary overflow may be due to several causes and is not well categorized. As can be seen in Table 6-2, disorders of tyrosine metabolism may result from either inherited or metabolic defects. Also, since two reactions are directly involved in the metabolism of tyrosine, the urine may contain excess tyrosine or its degradation products, *p*-hydroxyphenylpyruvic acid and *p*-hydroxyphenyllactic acid. Most frequently seen is a transitory tyrosinemia in premature infants, which is caused by underdevelopment of the liver function necessary to complete the tyrosine metabolism.[32] This condition seldom results in permanent damage, but it may be confused with PKU when urinary screening tests are performed on newborns, because the ferric chloride test will produce a green color. However, this reaction can be distinguished from the PKU reaction with ferric chloride because the green color fades rapidly. Acquired severe liver disease also will produce tyrosyluria resembling that of the transitory newborn variety and, of course, is a more serious condition. In both instances, rarely seen tyrosine and leucine crystals may be observed

TABLE 6-3. Summary of Urinary Screening Tests[23,31,41]

Test	Disorder	Observation
Color	Homogentisic Acid	Black
	Melanuria	Black
	Indicanuria	Dark Blue
	Porphyrinuria	Port Wine
Odor	Phenylketonuria	Mousy
	Maple Syrup Urine Disease	Maple Syrup
	Cystinuria	Sulfur
	Cystinosis	Sulfur
	Homocystinuria	Sulfur
Crystals	Tyrosyluria	Sheaths of fine needles
	Cystinuria	Colorless hexagonal plates
Ferric Chloride Tube Test	Phenylketonuria	Blue-Green
	Tyrosyluria	Transient Green
	Homogentisic Acid	Transient Blue
	Melanuria	Gray-Black
	Maple Syrup Urine Disease	Gray-Green
	Indicanuria	Violet-Blue with Chloroform
	5-HIAA	Blue-Green
Phenistix	Phenylketonuria	Gray-Green
	Tyrosyluria	Transient Green
Nitroso-naphthol	Phenylketonuria	Red
	Tyrosyluria	Red
	Maple Syrup Urine Disease	Red
	5-HIAA	Violet with Nitric Acid
2,4-Dinitrophenylhydrazine (DNPH)	Phenylketonuria	Yellow-White
	Tyrosyluria	Yellow-White
	Maple Syrup Urine Disease	Yellow-White
Cyanide-nitroprusside	Cystinuria	Red-Purple
	Cystinosis	Red-Purple
	Homocystinuria	Red-Purple
Silver-nitroprusside	Homocystinuria	Red-Purple
Ehrlich's Reaction	Porphyrinuria	Red
	Melanuria	Red
Acid-albumin Turbidity Test	Mucopolysaccharides	White Turbidity
Cetyltrimethylammonium Bromide (CTAB)	Mucopolysaccharides	White Turbidity

TABLE 6-3. *Continued*

Test	Disorder	Observation
Reducing Substances	Homogentisic Acid	Orange-Red
	Cystinosis	Orange-Red
	Melituria	Orange-Red

during microscopic examination of the urine sediment. Hereditary disorders in which enzymes required in the metabolic pathway are not produced present a serious and usually fatal condition that results in both liver and renal disease and in the appearance of a generalized aminoaciduria.[24]

The recommended urinary screening tests for tyrosine and its metabolites are the nitroso-naphthol test and the Millon test. Like the ferric chloride test, the nitroso-naphthol test is nonspecific and will react with compounds other than tyrosine and its metabolites. However, the presence of an orange-red color shows a positive reaction and indicates that further testing is needed. Millon's test will produce a red color in the presence of tyrosine or *p*-hydroxyphenylpyruvic acid. But because Millon's reagent contains the toxic substance mercury, the test is seldom performed in the routine clinical laboratory.

ALKAPTONURIA

Alkaptonuria was one of the six original "inborn errors of metabolism" described by Garrod in 1902. The name alkaptonuria was derived from the observation that urine from patients with this condition darkens after becoming alkaline from standing at room temperature. Therefore, the term "alkali lover," or alkaptonuria, was adopted. This metabolic defect is actually the third major one in the phenylalanine-tyrosine pathway and consists of failure to inherit the gene to produce the enzyme homogentisic acid oxidase. Without this enzyme, the phenylalanine-tyrosine pathway cannot proceed to completion, and homogentisic acid accumulates in the blood, tissues, and urine. This condition does not usually manifest itself clinically in early childhood. But in later life, brown pigment becomes deposited in the body tissues and may eventually lead to arthritis.[11] A high percentage of persons with alkaptonuria develop liver and cardiac disorders.[39]

Homogentisic acid will react in several of the routinely used screening tests for metabolic disorders, including the ferric chloride test, in which a transient deep blue color is produced in the tube test and a negative reaction occurs with Phenistix.[23] A yellow precipitate is produced in the Benedict's test or Clinitest, indicating the presence of a reducing substance. A more specific screening test for urinary homogentisic acid is to add alkali to freshly voided urine and observe for darkening of the color; however, large amounts of ascorbic acid will interfere with this reaction.[41] The addition of silver nitrate and ammonium hydroxide will also produce a black urine. A spectrophotometric method to obtain quantitative measurements of both urine and plasma homogentisic acid is also available.[36]

MELANURIA

We have been discussing the phenylalanine-tyrosine metabolic pathway illustrated in Figure 6-1; however, as is the case with many amino acids, a second metabolic pathway also exists for tyrosine. This pathway is responsible for production of melanin, thyroxine, epinephrine, protein, and tyrosine-sulfate.[24] Of these substances, the major concern of the urinalysis laboratory is melanin, the pigment responsible for the color of hair, skin, and eyes. Deficient production of melanin results in albinism.

Like homogentisic acid, increased urinary melanin will produce a darkening of urine when it is exposed to air. Elevation of urinary melanin is a serious finding that indicates the overproliferation of the normal melanin producing cells (malignant melanoma). These tumors secrete a colorless precursor of melanin, 5,6-dihydroxyindole, that oxidizes to melanogen and then to melanin, producing the characteristic dark urine. Differentiation between the presence of melanin and homogentisic acid must certainly be made.

Melanin will react with ferric chloride, sodium nitroprusside, and Ehrlich's reagent.[1] In the ferric chloride tube test, a gray or black precipitate will form in the presence of melanin and is easily differentiated from the transient blue-green color produced by homogentisic acid. Although it is not specific for melanin, the nitroprusside test is a frequently performed screening procedure. A red color is produced by the reaction of melanin and sodium nitroprusside. Interference due to red color from acetone and creatinine can be avoided by adding glacial acetic acid, which will cause melanin to revert to a green-black color, whereas acetone turns purple, and creatinine becomes amber.[3]

SUMMARY OF URINE SCREENING TESTS FOR DISORDERS OF THE PHENYLALANINE-TYROSINE PATHWAY

PHENYLKETONURIA

1. Phenistix
2. Ferric chloride tube test

TYROSYLURIA

1. Nitroso-naphthol test
2. Millon's test

ALKAPTONURIA

1. Ferric chloride tube test
2. Benedict's test or Clinitest
3. Alkalization of fresh urine

MELANURIA

1. Ferric chloride tube test
2. Sodium nitroprusside test
3. Ehrlich's test

MAPLE SYRUP URINE DISEASE

Although this is a rare disease, a brief discussion is included in this chapter because the urinalysis laboratory can provide valuable information for the essential early detection of this disease.

Maple syrup urine disease is referred to as a disorder of the branched chain amino acids produced by an inborn error of metabolism, inherited as an autosomal recessive. The amino acids involved are leucine, isoleucine, and valine. The metabolic pathway begins normally, with the transamination of the three amino acids in the liver to the keto acids α-ketoisovaleric, α-ketoisocaproic, and α-keto-β-methylvaleric. However, failure to inherit the gene for the enzyme necessary to produce oxidative decarboxylation of these keto acids results in their accumulation in the blood and urine.[13]

Newborns with maple syrup urine disease begin to exhibit clinical symptoms associated with failure to thrive after approximately 1 week. The presence of the disease may be suspected from these clinical symptoms; however, many other conditions have similar symptoms. Due to the rapid accumulation of keto acids in the urine, the disease may be detected by personnel in the urinalysis laboratory through the observation of a specimen that produces a strong odor resembling maple syrup. Even though a report of urine odor is not part of the routine urinalysis, notifying the physician about this unusual finding can prevent the development of severe mental retardation and even death. Current studies have shown that if maple syrup urine disease is detected by the

11th day, the disorder can be controlled by dietary regulation and careful monitoring of urinary keto acid concentrations.[6]

The screening test most frequently performed for keto acids is the 2,4-dinitrophenylhydrazine (DNPH) reaction. Addition of DNPH to urine that contains keto acids will produce a yellow turbidity or precipitate. The DNPH test can also be used for home monitoring of diagnosed cases. Large doses of ampicillin will interfere with the DNPH reaction, and as would be expected, the ferric chloride test will also be positive. Like many other urinary screening tests, the DNPH reaction is not specific for maple syrup urine disease, since keto acids are present in other disorders, including phenylketonuria. However, treatment can be started on the basis of odor, clinical symptoms, and a positive DNPH test, while confirmatory procedures using amino acid chromatography and measurement of the decarboxylase activity in the patient's leukocytes are being performed.[40] Studies have also recently shown that heterozygote carriers of the defective gene can be detected using the leukocyte decarboxylase test.[5]

TRYPTOPHAN METABOLISM DISORDERS

The major concern of the urinalysis laboratory in the metabolism of tryptophan is the increased urinary excretion of the metabolites indican and 5-hydroxyindoleacetic acid (5-HIAA). Figure 6-3 shows a simplified diagram of the metabolic pathways by which these substances are produced. Other metabolic pathways of tryptophan are not included because they do not relate directly to the urinalysis laboratory.

INDICAN

Under normal conditions, most of the tryptophan that enters the intestine is either reabsorbed for use by the body in the production of protein or is converted to indole by the intestinal bacteria and excreted in the feces.[28] However, in certain intestinal disorders (including obstruction, the presence of abnormal bacteria, malabsorption syndromes, and a rare inherited disorder, Hartnup disease), increased amounts of tryptophan are converted to indole. The indole is then reabsorbed and circulated to the liver, where it is converted to indican and then excreted in the urine. Indican excreted in the urine is colorless until oxidized by exposure to air to form the dye indigo blue. Early diagnosis of this disorder of tryptophan metabolism is sometimes made when mothers report a blue staining of their infant's diapers, referred to as the "blue diaper syndrome."[8] Urinary indican will react with acidic ferric chloride to form a deep blue or violet color that can subsequently be extracted into chloroform.[3]

Except in cases of Hartnup disease, correction of the underlying intestinal disorder will return urinary indican levels to normal. The inherited defect in Hartnup disease affects not only the intestinal reabsorption of tryptophan, but also the renal tubular reabsorption of other amino acids, resulting in a generalized aminoaciduria. The defective renal transport of amino acids does not appear to affect other renal tubular functions. Therefore, with proper dietary supplements, persons with Hartnup disease have a good prognosis.[20]

5-HYDROXYINDOLEACETIC ACID

As shown in Figure 6-3, a second metabolic pathway of tryptophan is for the production of serotonin utilized in the stimulation of smooth muscles. Serotonin is produced from tryptophan by the argentaffin cells in the intestine and is carried through the body primarily by the platelets. Normally, most of the serotonin is used by the body; only small amounts of its degradation product, 5-hydroxyindoleacetic acid (5-HIAA), are available for excretion in the urine. However, when malignant tumors involving the argentaffin cells develop, excess amounts of serotonin are produced, resulting in the elevation of urinary 5-HIAA levels.

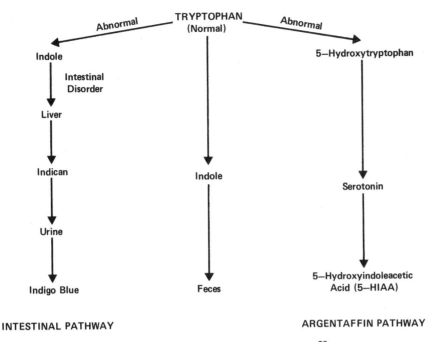

TRYPTOPHAN
(Normal)

Abnormal   Abnormal

Indole   5–Hydroxytryptophan

Intestinal
Disorder

Liver

Indican   Indole

Urine

Indigo Blue   Feces

Serotonin

5–Hydroxyindoleacetic
Acid (5–HIAA)

INTESTINAL PATHWAY   ARGENTAFFIN PATHWAY

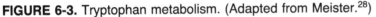

FIGURE 6-3. Tryptophan metabolism. (Adapted from Meister.[28])

The addition of nitrous acid and 1-nitroso-2-naphthol to urine that contains 5-HIAA causes the appearance of a purple to black color, depending on the amount of 5-HIAA present. The normal daily excretion of 5-HIAA is 2 to 8 mg, and argentaffin cell tumors will produce from 160 to 628 mg per 24 hours.[37] Therefore, the test is usually performed on a random or first morning specimen because there can be little chance of false-negative results. If a 24-hour sample is used, it must be preserved with hydrochloric acid. Patients must be given explicit dietary instructions prior to the collection of any sample to be tested for 5-HIAA, because serotonin is a major constituent of foods such as bananas, pineapples, and tomatoes. Interference will also be caused by medications, including phenothiazines and acetanilids.[37]

CYSTINE METABOLISM DISORDERS

There are two distinct disorders of cystine metabolism that exhibit renal manifestations. Confusion as to their relationship existed for many years following the discovery by Wollaston in 1810 of renal calculi consisting of cystine.[18] It is now known that although both disorders are inherited, one is a defect in the renal tubular transport of amino acids (cystinuria) and the other is an inborn error of metabolism (cystinosis).

CYSTINURIA

As the name implies, this condition is characterized by elevated amounts of the amino acid cystine in the urine. The presence of increased urinary cystine is not due to a defect in the metabolism of cystine, but rather to the inability of the renal tubules to reabsorb cystine filtered by the glomerulus. The demonstration that not only cystine, but also lysine, arginine, and ornithine are not reabsorbed has ruled out the possibility of an error in metabolism even though the condition is inherited.[7] The disorder has two modes of inheritance: one in which reabsorption of all four amino acids, cystine, lysine, arginine, and ornithine, is affected; and the other condition in which only cystine and lysine are not reabsorbed. The primary clinical consideration in cystinuria is the tendency of persons with defective reabsorption of all four amino acids to form calculi.

Approximately 65 percent of these people can be expected to produce calculi early in life.[18]

Because cystine is much less soluble than the other three amino acids, laboratory screening determinations are based on the observation of cystine crystals in the sediment of concentrated or first morning specimens. Cystine is also the only amino acid found during the analysis of calculi from these patients. Elevations in the other three amino acids must be determined separately using chromatography procedures. A chemical screening test for urinary cystine can be performed using cyanide-nitroprusside. Reduction of cystine by sodium cyanide followed by the addition of nitroprusside will produce a red-purple color in a specimen that contains excess cystine. False-positive reactions will occur in the presence of ketones and homocystine, and additional tests that are specific for these substances may have to be performed to rule them out.

CYSTINOSIS

Regarded as a genuine inborn error of metabolism, cystinosis can occur in three variations ranging from a severe fatal disorder developed in infancy to a benign form appearing in adulthood. The incomplete metabolism of cystine results in crystalline deposits of cystine in many areas of the body, including the cornea, bone marrow, lymph nodes, and internal organs.[34] A major defect in the renal tubular reabsorption mechanism, referred to as the Fanconi syndrome, also occurs. Patients exhibit the inability to reabsorb amino acids, phosphorous, potassium, sugars, and water. Routine laboratory findings include polyuria, generalized aminoaciduria, positive tests for reducing substances, and lack of urinary concentration. In severe cases, there is a gradual progression to total renal failure.[35]

HOMOCYSTINURIA

Defects in the metabolism of homocystine can have major clinical significance, since excessive accumulation of homocystine may be the second most common metabolic disorder producing mental retardation.[38] As mentioned earlier, increased urinary homocystine gives a positive result with the cyanide-nitroprusside test. Therefore, laboratory screening for homocystinuria can be performed by following a positive cyanide-nitroprusside test with a silver-nitroprusside test, in which only homocystine will react. The use of silver nitrate in place of sodium cyanide will reduce homocystine to its nitroprusside-reactive form but will not reduce cystine. Consequently, a positive reaction in the silver-nitroprusside test confirms the presence of homocystinuria.[41]

PORPHYRIN DISORDERS

Porphyrins are the intermediate compounds in the production of heme. The basic pathway for heme synthesis is illustrated in Figure 6-4. As can be seen, there are a number of stages at which production can be disrupted. The major disorders of porphyrin metabolism and the sites at which they interrupt the pathway are also shown in Figure 6-4.[29] Blockage of a pathway reaction will result in an accumulation of the product formed just prior to the interruption. Detection and identification of this compound in the urine serves as an aid to the diagnosis of the particular disorder. Conditions that result in the appearance of porphyrinuria are collectively termed porphyrias and can be inherited as inborn errors of metabolism or acquired through erythrocytic and hepatic malfunctions caused either by metabolic disease or exposure to toxic agents. Lead poisoning is the most common cause of porphyrinuria. The individual porphyrias will not be discussed separately in this section, and many varieties other than those shown in Figure 6-4 also exist.[9] Diagnosis of these other types often requires analysis of feces and erythrocytes; whereas the porphyrias shown in Figure 6-4 are more closely associated with the analysis of urine.

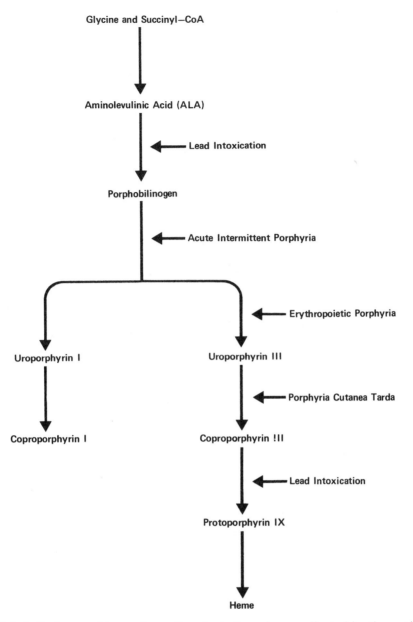

Glycine and Succinyl—CoA

Aminolevulinic Acid (ALA)

← Lead Intoxication

Porphobilinogen

← Acute Intermittent Porphyria

← Erythropoietic Porphyria

Uroporphyrin I   Uroporphyrin III

← Porphyria Cutanea Tarda

Coproporphyrin I   Coproporphyrin III

← Lead Intoxication

Protoporphyrin IX

Heme

FIGURE 6-4. Pathway of heme formation, including stages affected by the major disorders of porphyrin metabolism. (Adapted from Miale.[29])

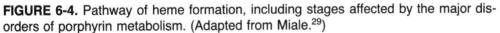

A possible indication of the presence of porphyrinuria is the observation of a red or port-wine color to the urine. However, porphobilinogen is excreted as a colorless compound, and the color change will not occur unless the urine is acidic and remains exposed to air for several hours. As we have seen with other inherited disorders, the presence of congenital porphyria is sometimes suspected from a red discoloration of infants' diapers.[43]

The two screening tests for porphyrinuria utilize the Ehrlich reaction and fluorescence under ultraviolet light from a Wood's lamp. The Ehrlich reaction can only be used for the detection of aminolevulinic acid (ALA) and porphobilinogen; the fluorescent technique must be used for the other porphyrins. The Ehrlich reaction, including the Watson-Schwartz test for differentiation between the presence of urobilinogen and porphobilinogen, was discussed in detail in Chapter 4. A more rapid method for the detection of increased porphobilinogen that does not require a separation phase is the Hoesch test. It is most valuable for patients suspected of having acute attacks of porphyria and is performed by adding only two drops of urine to 1 or 2 milliliters of Ehrlich's reagent and observing for the appearance of a red color at the top of the solution.[25] When using the Ehrlich reaction to measure increased ALA, acetylacetone must be added to the specimen to convert the ALA to porphobilinogen prior to performing the Ehrlich test.[26] The detection of increased levels of urinary ALA is a primary screening test for lead poisoning. Mass screening programs often supply cation exchange paper dipsticks for the collection of specimens. The dipstick is allowed to dry and is mailed to the laboratory, where the ALA is eluted from the paper and tested.[17]

Fluorescent screening for the other porphyrins requires their extraction into a mixture of glacial acetic acid and ethyl acetate. The solvent layer is then examined under a Wood's lamp. Negative reactions have a faint blue fluorescence. Positive reactions will fluoresce as pink, violet, or red, depending upon the concentration of porphyrins. If the presence of interfering substances is suspected, the organic layer can be removed to a separate tube and 0.5 ml of hydrochloric acid added to the tube. Only porphyrins will be extracted into the acid layer, which will then produce a bright orange-red fluorescence. The fluorescence method will not distinguish among uroporphyrin, coproporphyrin, and protoporphyrin unless specimens are subjected to changes in pH, but will rule out porphobilinogen and aminolevulinic acid.[16] The identification of the specific porphyrins requires additional extraction techniques and, possibly, analysis of fecal and erythrocyte samples.

SUMMARY OF PORPHYRIN SCREENING TESTS

EHRLICH'S REACTION
1. Aminolevulinic acid
2. Porphobilinogen

ULTRAVIOLET LIGHT
1. Uroporphyrin
2. Coproporphyrin
3. Protoporphyrin

MUCOPOLYSACCHARIDE DISORDERS

Mucopolysaccharides, or glycosaminoglycans, are a group of large compounds located primarily in the connective tissue. They consist of a protein core with numerous polysaccharide branches. Inherited disorders of the metabolism of these compounds prevent the complete breakdown of the polysaccharide portion of the compounds, resulting in the accumulation of the incompletely metabolized polysaccharide portions in the lysosomes of the connective tissue cells and their increased excretion in the urine.[41] The products most frequently found in the urine are dermatan sulfate, keratan sulfate, and heparan sulfate, with the appearance of a particular substance being determined by the specific metabolic error that was inherited. Therefore, identification of the specific degradation product present may be necessary to establish a specific diagnosis.[27] There are many types of mucopolysaccharidoses, but the best known are Hurler's syndrome, Hunter's syndrome, and Sanfilippo's syndrome. In both Hurler's and Hunter's syndromes, the skeletal structure is abnormal and there is severe mental retardation; in Hurler's syndrome, mucopolysaccharides accumulate in the cornea of the eye. Both syndromes are usually fatal during childhood; whereas in Sanfilippo's syndrome, the only abnormality is mental retardation.[42]

Urinary screening tests for mucopolysaccharides are requested either as part of a routine battery of tests performed on all newborns or on infants who exhibit symptoms of mental retardation or failure to thrive. The most frequently used screening tests are the acid-albumin and cetyltrimethylammonium bromide (CTAB) turbidity tests and the metachromatic staining spot tests. In both the acid-albumin and the CTAB tests, a thick, white turbidity will form when these reagents are added to urine that contains mucopolysaccharides. Turbidity is usually graded on a scale of 0 to 4 after 10 minutes with acid-albumin and after 30 minutes with CTAB. Consequently, the acid-albumin procedure is recommended for mass screening programs.[4] Metachromatic staining procedures use basic dyes to react with the acidic mucopolysaccharides. MPS papers (Ames Company, Elkhart, Indiana) contain Azure A dye, and urine that contains mucopolysaccharides will produce a blue spot that cannot be washed away by a dilute acidified methanol solution.[12]

OTHER SCREENING TESTS
COPPER REDUCTION TESTS

Discussed previously in Chapter 4, the Benedict's and Clinitest copper reduction tests are included again in this section because they are usually included in newborn screening programs. The presence of increased urinary sugar (melituria) is most frequently due to an inherited disorder. In fact, pentosuria was one of Garrod's original six inborn errors of metabolism.[14] Fortunately, the majority of meliturias cause no disturbance to body metabolism.[19] However, when a positive test for urinary reducing substances is encountered, the specimen must be screened for the presence of galactose or fructose, because disorders in the metabolism of these sugars do cause serious pathologic conditions.

SULKOWITCH'S TEST

Historically, the Sulkowitch test was used as a qualitative measurement of urinary calcium. Sulkowitch's reagent (which contains oxalic acid, ammonium oxalate, and glacial acetic acid) reacts with urinary calcium, creating turbidity due to the precipitation of calcium oxalate. Turbidity is graded on a scale of 0 to 4. It is now accepted that a qualitative measurement of urinary calcium provides little useful diagnostic information, and urinary calcium in conjunction with serum calcium is quantitatively measured in the chemistry laboratory.

SUMMARY

A summary of urinary screening tests is presented in Table 6-3.

REFERENCES

1. BEELER, MF AND HENRY, JB: *Melanogenuria: Evaluation of several commonly used laboratory procedures.* JAMA 176:52–54, 1961.
2. BRADLEY, GM: *Urinary screening tests in the infant and young child.* Hum Pathol 2(2):309–320, 1971.
3. BRADLEY, M AND SCHUMANN, GB: Examination of the urine. In HENRY, JB (ED): *Clinical Diagnosis and Management by Laboratory Methods.* WB Saunders, Philadelphia, 1984.
4. CARTER, CH, WAN, AT, AND CARPENTER, DG: *Commonly used tests in the detection of Hurler's syndrome.* J Pediatr 73:217–221, 1968.
5. CHUANG, DT, ET AL: *Detection of heterozygotes in MSUD: Measurement of branched-chain α-ketoacid dehydrogenase and its components in cell cultures.* Am J Hum Genet 34(3):416–424, 1982.
6. CLOW, CL, READE, TH, AND SCRIVER, CR: *Outcome of early and long-term management of classical maple syrup urine disease.* Pediatrics 68(6):856–862, 1981.

7. CRAWHILL, JC: *Cystinuria: Diagnosis and treatment.* In NYHAN, WL (ED): *Heritable Disorders of Amino Acids.* John Wiley & Sons, New York, 1974.

8. DRUMMOND, KN, ET AL: *The blue diaper syndrome:Familial hypercalcemia.* Am J Med 37:928–948, 1964.

9. EADES, L: *The porphyrins and porphyrias.* Annu Rev Med 12:251–270, 1961.

10. EFFRON, ML: *Aminoaciduria.* N Engl J Med 272:1058–1067, 1965.

11. FLANAGEN, SM: *Urinalysis Problem.* Am J Med Technol 48(5):375–376, 1982.

12. FREE, AH AND FREE, HM: *Urodynamics: Concepts Relating to Routine Urine Chemistry.* Ames Co, Division of Miles Laboratories, Elkhart, Indiana, 1978.

13. FRIMPTON, GW: *Aminoacidurias due to inherited disorders of metabolism.* N Engl J Med 1289:835–901, 1973.

14. GARROD, AE: *Inborn Errors of Metabolism.* Henry Froude & Hodder & Stoughton, London, 1923.

15. GUTHRIE, R: *Blood screening for phenylketonuria.* JAMA 178(8):863, 1961.

16. HAINING, RG, HULSE, T, AND LABBE, RF: *Rapid porphyrin screening of urine, stool and blood.* Clin Chem 16(6):460–466, 1961.

17. HANKIN, L, ET AL: *Simplified method for mass screening for lead poisoning based on α-aminolevulinic acid in urine.* Clin Pediatr 9:707, 1970.

18. HARRIS, H AND ROBSON, EB: *Cystinuria.* Am J Med 22:774–783, 1957.

19. HIATT, HH: *Pentosuria.* In STANBURY, JB, WYNGAARDEN, JB, AND FREDRICKSON, DS (EDS): *The Metabolic Basis of Inherited Diseases.* McGraw-Hill, New York, 1978.

20. JEPSON, JB: *Hartnup's disease.* In STANBURY, JB, WYNGAARDEN, JB, AND FREDRICKSON, DS (EDS): *The Metabolic Basis of Inherited Diseases.* McGraw-Hill, New York, 1978.

21. KIRKMAN, H, ET AL: *Fifteen year experience with screening for phenylketonuria with an automated fluorometric method.* Am J Hum Genet 34(5):743–752, 1982.

22. KISHEL, M AND LIGHTY, P: *Some diaper brands give false-positive tests for PKU.* N Engl J Med 300(4):200, 1979.

23. KNIGHT, JA AND WU, JT: *Screening profile for detection of inherited metabolic disorders.* Laboratory Medicine 13(11):681–687, 1982.

24. KRETCHMER, N AND ETZWILER, DD: *Disorders associated with the metabolism of phenylalanine and tyrosine.* Pediatrics 21:445–475, 1958.

25. LAMON, J, WITH, TK, AND REDEKER, AG: *The Hoesch test: Bedside screening for urinary porphobilinogen in patients with suspected porphyria.* Clin Chem 20:1438–1440, 1974.

26. MAUZERALL, D AND GRANICK, S: *The occurrence and determination of D-amino-levulinic acid and porphobilinogen in urine.* J Biol Chem 219:435–436, 1956.

27. MCKUSICK, VA, NEUFELD, EF, AND KELLY, TE: *The mucopolysaccharide storage diseases.* In STANBURY, JB, WYNGAARDEN, JB, AND FREDRICKSON, DS (EDS): *The Metabolic Basis of Inherited Diseases.* McGraw-Hill, New York, 1978.

28. MEISTER, A: *Biochemistry of the Amino Acids.* Academic Press, New York, 1965.

29. MIALE, JB: *Laboratory Medicine: Hematology.* CV Mosby, St. Louis, 1982.

30. PANKAU, EF: *Purple urine bags.* J Urol 130(2):372–373, 1983.

31. PERRY, TL, HANSEN, SH, AND MACDOUGALL, L: *Urinary screening tests in the prevention of mental deficiency.* Can Med Assoc J 95:89–97, 1966.

32. RACE, GJ AND WHITE, MG: *Basic Urinalysis.* Harper & Row, Hagerstown, Maryland, 1979.

33. RAGSDALE, N AND KOCH, R: *Phenylketonuria: Detection and therapy.* Am J Nurs 64:90–96, 1964.

34. SCHNEIDER, JA: *Recent advances in cystinosis.* In NYHAN, WL (ED): *Heritable Disorders of Amino Acids.* John Wiley & Sons, New York, 1974.

35. SCHNEIDER, JA, SCHULMAN, JD, AND SEEGMILLER, JE: *Cystinosis and the Fanconi syndrome.* In NYHAN, WL (ED): *Heritable Disorders of Amino Acids.* John Wiley & Sons, New York, 1974.

36. SEEGMILLER, JE, ET AL: *An enzymatic spectrophotometric method for the determination of homogentisic acid in plasma and urine.* J Biol Chem 236:774–777, 1961.
37. SJOERDSMA, A, WEISSBACH, H, AND UDENFRIEND, S: *Simple test for diagnosis of metastatic carcinoid (argentaffinoma).* JAMA 159(4):397, 1955.
38. SPAETH, GL AND BARBER, GW: *Prevalence of homocystinuria among the mentally retarded: Evaluation of a screening test.* Pediatrics 40:586–589, 1967.
39. STANBURY, JB: *The Metabolic Basis of Inherited Diseases.* McGraw-Hill, New York, 1964.
40. SYNDERMON, SE: *Patterns of clinical expression and genetic variations.* In NYHAN, WL (ED): *Heritable Disorders of Amino Acids.* John Wiley & Sons, New York, 1974.
41. THOMAS, GH AND HOWELL, RR: *Selected Screening Tests for Metabolic Diseases.* Yearbook Medical Publishers, Chicago, 1973.
42. THOMPSON, JS AND THOMPSON, MW: *Genetics in Medicine.* WB Saunders, Philadelphia, 1978.
43. WALDENSTROM, J: *The porphyrias as inborn errors of metabolism.* Am J Med 22:758–773, 1957.

STUDY QUESTIONS (Choose one best answer)

1. The appearance of abnormal metabolites in the urine due to a defect categorized as an "overflow type" may be caused by all of the following except:

   a. inborn errors of metabolism
   b. serum concentrations exceeding the tubular reabsorption capability
   c. abnormalities in the tubular reabsorption mechanism
   d. disruption of normal enzyme function due to exposure to toxic substances

2. Phenylketonuria is caused by:

   a. excessive ingestion of milk products containing phenylalanine
   b. inability to metabolize tyrosine
   c. lack of the enzyme phenylalanine hydroxylase
   d. a mousy odor in the urine

3. Initial screening for PKU performed on newborns prior to their discharge from the hospital utilizes a blood sample rather than a urine sample because:

   a. urine samples are more difficult to collect
   b. blood is routinely collected on all newborns for other tests
   c. it is easier to measure phenylalanine than phenylpyruvic acid
   d. increased serum phenylalanine occurs earlier than increased urine phenylpyruvic acid

4. The Guthrie test is:

   a. a bacterial inhibition test
   b. a fluorometric procedure
   c. a chemical procedure measured by spectrophotometer
   d. a bacterial agglutination test

5. Detection of urine phenylpyruvic acid by Phenistix utilizes a chemical reaction between phenylpyruvic acid and:

   a. sodium chloride
   b. ferric chloride
   c. phenylalanine
   d. *Bacillus subtilis*

6. The color of a positive PKU reaction on Phenistix is:

   a. yellow-orange
   b. red-orange
   c. gray-green
   d. brown-black

7. A transient positive reaction on Phenistix may indicate:

   a. deterioration of the test strip
   b. reduced levels of phenylpyruvic acid
   c. the presence of phenylalanine
   d. tyrosine and its metabolites

8. The abnormal metabolite that is present in the urine in alkaptonuria is:

   a. homogentisic acid
   b. alkaptonpyruvate
   c. phenylpyruvate
   d. tyrosine

9. A routine urinalysis is performed on a specimen that has turned dark after standing in the lab. The urine is acidic and has negative chemical tests except for the appearance of a red color on the ketone area of the dipstick. One should suspect:

   a. phenylketonuria
   b. diabetic ketosis
   c. alkaptonuria
   d. melanuria

10. Although urine odor is not included in the routine urinalysis, it can be important in the early detection of:

    a. branched chain amino acid disorders
    b. straight chain amino acid disorders
    c. all amino acid disorders
    d. no medically important amino acid disorders

11. Confirmation of maple syrup urine disease is made on the basis of:

    a. urine odor
    b. positive 2,4-dinitrophenylhydrazine test
    c. positive ferric chloride test
    d. amino acid chromatography

12. Analysis of urine from an infant whose mother reported a blue staining on the diapers showed increased levels of indican and a generalized aminoaciduria. On the basis of these findings, the infant was diagnosed as having:

    a. an intestinal obstruction
    b. a protein malabsorption syndrome
    c. Fanconi's syndrome
    d. Hartnup disease

13. Under normal conditions, tryptophan that is not reabsorbed in the intestine is removed from the body as:

    a. indican in the urine
    b. indole in the liver
    c. indole in the feces
    d. serotonin in the urine

14. The finding of increased amounts of the serotonin degradation product 5-hydroxy-indoleacetic acid in the urine is indicative of:

    a. platelet disorders
    b. intestinal obstruction
    c. malabsorption syndromes
    d. argentaffin cell tumors

15. Interference will occur in 5-HIAA tests if patients are not properly instructed in:

    a. specimen collection procedures
    b. dietary restrictions
    c. time of specimen collection
    d. coordination of blood and urine samples

16. Place the appropriate letter in front of the statement that best matches the condition:

    a. Cystinuria   b. Cystinosis
    ____ true inborn error of metabolism
    ____ defective reabsorption of cystine, lysine, ornithine, and arginine
    ____ tendency to form renal calculi
    ____ Fanconi's syndrome
    ____ generalized aminoaciduria

17. Chemical screening tests for cystine will produce false-positive results in the presence of urinary ketones because:

    a. cystine is not reduced by sodium cyanide
    b. cystine should only be tested using chromatography
    c. the test reagent is nitroprusside
    d. glucose present in diabetic ketosis concentrates the specimen

18. Porphyrins are intermediary compounds in the formation of:

    a. amino acids
    b. serotonin
    c. heme
    d. bilirubin

19. The presence of porphobilinogen in the urine can be suspected when:

   a. acidic urine turns a port-wine color after standing
   b. alkaline urine turns a port-wine color after standing
   c. freshly excreted urine is acidic and port wine in color
   d. freshly excreted urine is alkaline and port wine in color

20. Urine from a child suspected of having lead poisoning has a red fluorescence under a Wood's lamp. This finding is:

   a. inconsistent with lead poisoning because aminolevulinic acid does not fluoresce
   b. consistent with lead poisoning because coproporphyrin fluoresces under ultra-violet light
   c. only consistent with lead poisoning if uroporphyrin is also increased
   d. only consistent if protoporphyrin can be demonstrated using Ehrlich's reagent

21. Hurler's and Sanfilippo's syndromes present with mental retardation and increased urinary:

   a. porphyrins
   b. amino acids
   c. maltose
   d. mucopolysaccharides

22. The presence of urinary reducing substances is of particular concern in:

   a. pregnant women
   b. newborns
   c. adolescent males
   d. menopausal women

23. The Sulkowitch test screens for urinary:

   a. glucose
   b. oxalate
   c. calcium
   d. ammonia

CASE STUDIES

1. During a 2-week vacation in Hawaii, Tom Richardson develops stomach pains. Immediately upon his return, he visits his physician, who orders a chemistry profile, urine 5-HIAA, and an upper GI series. All tests are normal except the 5-HIAA, and Mr. Richardson's stomach discomfort has ended.

   a. What could account for the elevated 5-HIAA?
   b. How can Tom's physician verify that he does not have a tumor of the argentaffin cells?

2. Bobby Williams, age 8, is admitted through the emergency department with a ruptured appendix. Although surgery is successful, Bobby's recovery is slow, and the physicians are concerned about his health prior to the ruptured appendix. Bobby's mother states that he has always been noticeably underweight despite a balanced diet and a strong appetite and that his younger brother exhibits similar characteris-

tics. A note in his chart from the first postoperative day reports that the evening nurse noticed a purple coloration to the urinary catheter bag.[30]

   a. Is the catheter bag color significant?
   b. What additional tests should be run?
   c. What condition can be suspected from this history?
   d. What is Bobby's prognosis?

3. Baby girl Miller receives the customary PKU test prior to her discharge from the hospital, and the result is negative. At her 6-week examination, the physician observes that she is lethargic and has failed to thrive. He orders a battery of metabolic screening tests. The ferric chloride tube test turns a gray-green-blue color, and a yellow-white precipitate forms with 2,4-dinitrophenylhydrazine. Negative reactions are found with cyanide-nitroprusside, acid-albumin, and Clinitest.

   a. What two conditions do these results suggest?
   b. What further testing could be done?
   c. Is the negative PKU test of any significance? Explain your answer.

7
CEREBROSPINAL FLUID

INSTRUCTIONAL OBJECTIVES

Upon completion of this chapter, readers will be able to:

1. list the three major functions of cerebrospinal fluid

2. distribute CSF specimen tubes numbered 1, 2, and 3 to their appropriate laboratory sections

3. describe the appearance of normal and infectious CSF

4. define xanthochromia and state its significance

5. differentiate between the appearance of a bloody specimen caused by a cerebral hemorrhage and one that resulted from a traumatic spinal tap

6. calculate CSF white and red blood cell counts when given the number of cells seen, amount of specimen dilution, and the squares counted in the Neubauer chamber

7. briefly explain the methods used to correct for white blood cells and protein that are artificially introduced during a traumatic tap

8. name the type of white blood cell primarily associated with bacterial, viral, tubercular, and parasitic meningitis

9. describe and give the significance of abnormal macrophages in the CSF

10. give two differences in the appearance of normal choroidal cells and malignant cells

11. state the normal value for CSF total protein

12. list three pathologic conditions that produce an elevated CSF protein

13. discuss the basic principles associated with the turbidimetric and the dye-binding methods of CSF protein analysis

14. state the normal CSF glucose value

15. name the possible pathologic significance of a decreased CSF glucose

16. briefly discuss the diagnostic value of CSF lactate, glutamine, and lactic dehydrogenase determinations

17. name the microorganism associated with a positive India ink preparation

18. state the diagnostic value of the Limulus Lysate test

19. determine if a suspected case of meningitis is most probably of bacterial,

viral, fungal, or tubercular origin, when presented with pertinent laboratory data

FORMATION AND PHYSIOLOGY

First recognized by Cotugno in 1764, cerebrospinal fluid (CSF) is the third major fluid of the body.[15] The CSF provides a physiologic system to supply nutrients to the nervous tissue and remove metabolic wastes, and a mechanical barrier to cushion the brain and spinal cord against trauma. Approximately 20 ml of fluid are produced every hour in the choroid plexuses and reabsorbed by the arachnoid villi to maintain a total volume of 140 to 170 ml in adults, and 10 to 60 ml in neonates.[32,25] Figure 7-1 depicts the flow of the cerebrospinal fluid through the brain and spinal column. Production of CSF in the choroid plexuses is by filtration under hydrostatic pressure across the choroidal capillary wall and active transport secretion by the choroidal epithelial cells. Tightly fitting junctions between the endothelial cells of the capillaries and the choroid plexuses restrict entry of macromolecules such as protein, insoluble lipids, and substances bound to serum proteins. The chemical composition of the fluid does not resemble an ultra-filtrate of plasma due to bidirectional active transport between the CSF, interstitial brain fluid, brain cells, and blood in the brain capillaries. The term blood-brain barrier is used to represent all of the bidirectional exchanges between the blood, CSF, and brain, replacing the older individual terms CSF-blood barrier, CSF-brain barrier, and blood-brain barrier.[10]

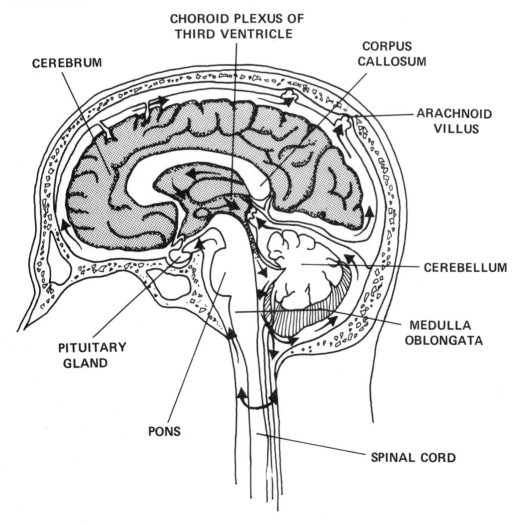

FIGURE 7-1. The flow of cerebrospinal fluid through the brain and spinal column.

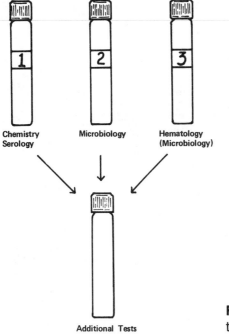

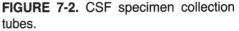

Chemistry
Serology

Microbiology

Hematology
(Microbiology)

Additional Tests

FIGURE 7-2. CSF specimen collection tubes.

SPECIMEN COLLECTION

Cerebrospinal fluid is routinely collected by lumbar puncture between the third, fourth, or fifth lumbar vertebrae. Although this is not a complicated procedure, it does require certain precautions, including measurement of the intracranial pressure and careful technique to prevent the introduction of infection or the damaging of neural tissue. Specimens are usually collected in three sterile tubes, labeled 1, 2, and 3 in the order in which they are withdrawn. Tube 1 is used for chemical and serologic tests; Tube 2 is used for microbiology; Tube 3 is used for the cell count, because it is the least likely to contain cells introduced by the spinal tap procedure. If possible, Tube 3 may also be used by microbiology prior to hematology, because it is less likely to contain skin contaminants. Supernatant fluid that is left over after each section has performed its tests may be used for additional chemical or serologic tests. Excess fluid should not be discarded until there is no further use for it (Fig. 7-2).

CSF IN THE HEMATOLOGY LABORATORY
APPEARANCE

The initial appearance of the normally crystal clear CSF can provide valuable diagnostic information (Table 7-1). Examination of the fluid occurs first at the bedside and is also included in the hematology report. The major terminology used to describe CSF appearance includes crystal clear, cloudy or turbid, milky, xanthochromic, and bloody. A cloudy, turbid, or milky specimen can be the result of an increased protein or lipid concentration, but it also may be indicative of infection, with the cloudiness being caused by the presence of white blood cells. All specimens, however, should be treated with extreme care because they can be highly contagious.

Xanthochromia is a term that is used to describe CSF supernatant that is either pink, orange, or yellow. A variety of factors can cause the appearance of xanthochromia, with the most common being the presence of red blood cell degradation products. Depending on the amount of blood and the length of time it has been present, the color

TABLE 7-1. Clinical Significance of CSF Appearance

Appearance	Cause	Major Significance
Crystal clear		Normal
Hazy, Turbid, Cloudy, Smoky, Milky	WBCs RBCs	Meningitis Hemorrhage Traumatic tap
	Microorganisms Protein	Meningitis Disorders that affect blood-brain barrier Production of IgG within CNS
Oily Bloody Xanthochromic	X-ray material RBCs Hemoglobin	Hemorrhage Old hemorrhage Lysed cells from traumatic tap
	Bilirubin	RBC breakdown Elevated serum bilirubin
	Merthiolate Carotene Protein	Contamination Increased serum levels SEE ABOVE
Clotted	Protein Clotting factors	SEE ABOVE Introduced by traumatic tap
Pellicle Formation	Protein Clotting factors	Tubercular meningitis

will vary from pink (very slight amount of oxyhemoglobin) to orange (heavy hemolysis) to yellow (conversion of oxyhemoglobin to unconjugated bilirubin). Other causes of xanthochromia include elevated serum bilirubin, presence of the pigment carotene, markedly increased protein concentrations, and melanoma pigment. Xanthochromia that is due to immature liver function is also commonly seen in infants, particularly in those who are premature.

TRAUMATIC COLLECTION

Grossly bloody CSF can be an indication of intracranial hemorrhage, but it may also be due to the puncture of a blood vessel during the spinal tap procedure. Three visual examinations of the collected specimens can usually determine whether the blood is the result of hemorrhage or "traumatic tap."

1. Uneven Distribution of Blood
   Blood from a cerebral hemorrhage will be evenly distributed throughout the three CSF specimen tubes; whereas a traumatic tap will have the heaviest concentration of blood in Tube 1, with gradually diminishing amounts in Tubes 2 and 3. Streaks of blood may also be seen in specimens acquired following a traumatic procedure.
2. Clot Formation
   Fluid collected from a traumatic tap may form clots due to the introduction of serum fibrinogen into the specimen. Bloody CSF caused by intracranial hemorrhage will not contain enough fibrinogen to clot. Diseases in which damage to the blood-brain barrier allows increased filtration of protein and coagulation factors will also cause clot formation. These conditions include meningitis, Froin's syndrome, and blockage of CSF circulation through the subarachnoid space.

A classic web-like pellicle is associated with tubercular meningitis and is frequently seen after overnight refrigeration of the fluid.[28]

3. Xanthochromic Supernatant

Red blood cells must usually remain in the CSF for approximately 2 hours before hemolysis begins; therefore, a xanthochromic supernatant would be the result of blood that has been present longer than that introduced by the traumatic tap. Care should be taken, however, to consider this examination in conjunction with those previously discussed since a very recent hemorrhage would produce a clear supernatant, and introduction of serum protein from a traumatic tap could also cause the fluid to appear xanthochromic. Microscopic examination of the fluid for the presence of crenated red blood cells, once considered an additional confirmation that blood was the result of intracranial hemorrhage, is not a reliable indication of hemorrhage and should not be used.[24]

CELL COUNT

The cell count that is routinely performed on CSF specimens is the leukocyte (WBC) count. As discussed earlier, the presence and significance of red blood cells can usually be ascertained from the appearance of the specimen. Therefore, red blood cell counts are usually performed only when a traumatic tap has occurred and it is necessary to correct for the leukocytes or protein introduced into the specimen. Any cell count should be performed immediately, because both white blood cells and red blood cells will begin to lyse within an hour.[13]

METHODOLOGY

Normal adult CSF contains 0 to 5 white blood cells per microliter. The number is higher in children, and as many as 30 mononuclear cells per microliter can be considered normal in newborns.[21] Specimens that contain up to 200 cells per microliter may appear clear, so it is necessary to microscopically examine all specimens.[12] Electronic counters cannot be used for CSF because of the variation in background counts and the possibility of falsely elevating normal or moderately high counts. Good correlation has been demonstrated between electronic and manual counts on specimens with over 1000 cells per microliter. However, the accepted method for CSF cell counts is to perform them manually in a counting chamber.[20] Either an improved Neubauer counting chamber (Fig. 7-3) or a Fuchs-Rosenthal chamber may be used. The procedures and calculations associated with the Neubauer chamber are discussed in this chapter.

Clear to slightly hazy specimens may be counted undiluted provided no overlapping of the cells is seen during the microscopic examination. Both chambers of the hemocytometer should be charged with fluid so that duplicate counts can be performed. When undiluted fluid is used, cells in all nine large squares of the chamber are counted (see Fig. 7-3). The number of cells per microliter is then calculated as follows:

$$\frac{\text{Number of Cells Counted} \times \text{Dilution (1)}}{\text{Number of Squares Counted (9)} \times \text{Volume of 1 Square (0.1)} \; \mu l}$$

This formula can be used for both diluted and undiluted specimens and offers flexibility in the number and size of the squares counted. Many varied calculations are available, including condensations of the formula to provide single factors by which to multiply the cell count. Keep in mind that the purpose of any calculation is to convert the number of cells counted in a specific amount of fluid to the number of cells that would be present in one microliter of fluid. Therefore, a factor can only be used when the dilution and counting area are specific for that factor. An example of a commonly used factor applies to the undiluted count discussed above. The formula can be condensed to read:

$$\text{Number of Cells Counted} \times \frac{1}{0.9} \text{ and then converted to}$$

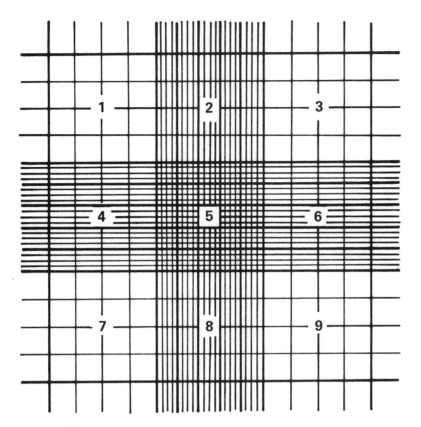

FIGURE 7-3. Neubauer counting chamber.

$$\text{Number of Cells Counted} \times \frac{10}{9} = \text{Cells/}\mu\text{l}$$

Sample calculations using both methods when 50 cells are counted would appear like this:

$$\frac{50 \text{ Cells} \times 1 \text{ (Dilution)}}{9 \text{ (Squares Counted)} \times 0.1 \ \mu\text{l (Volume per Square)}} = 56 \text{ Cells/}\mu\text{l}$$

$$50 \text{ Cells} \times \frac{10}{9} = 56 \text{ Cells/}\mu\text{l}$$

Dilutions of the CSF must be made when the specimen appears cloudy or, as stated above, when cells are too numerous to be accurately counted in an undiluted specimen. Diluting fluid (Turk's solution) for CSF white blood cell counts consists of 2 or 3 percent glacial acetic acid to lyse any red cells present and gentian violet to stain WBC nuclei, making the cells more prominent for counting. The most common dilutions are 1:10 and 1:20, depending on the turbidity of the fluid, and are prepared in Thoma WBC pipettes. The routine method of counting is the same as for blood counts, which is counting the cells in the four large corner squares (Fig. 7-4) and calculating the number of cells per microliter.

Example: 50 WBCs (from a CSF diluted 1:10) are counted in four large squares. Calculate the number of cells per microliter.

$$\frac{50 \text{ Cells} \times 10 \text{ (Dilution)}}{4 \text{ (Squares Counted)} \times 0.1 \ \mu\text{l (Volume per Square)}} = 1250 \text{ Cells/}\mu\text{l}$$

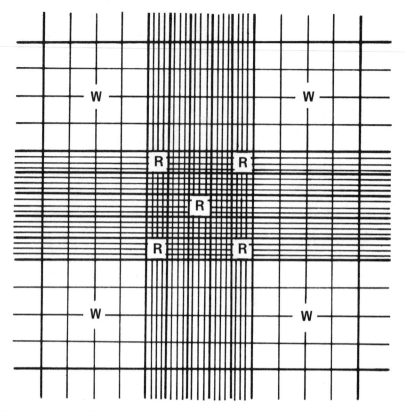

FIGURE 7-4. Areas of Neubauer counting chamber used for red and white cell counts.

RED BLOOD CELL COUNTS

Red blood cell counts on CSF are also performed by the same method used for blood counts and use routine red blood cell diluting fluid such as normal saline or Gowers' solution. Dilutions of 1:100 or 1:200, depending on the amount of blood present, are prepared in Thoma RBC pipettes. Cells are counted in the five small squares in the large center square (see Fig. 7-4), and the number of cells per microliter is calculated by the same basic formula used for WBC counts.

Example: 50 RBCs (from a CSF specimen resulting from a traumatic tap) are counted in five small squares. The dilution is 1:100. Calculate the number of cells per microliter.

$$\frac{50 \text{ Cells} \times 100 \text{ (Dilution)}}{5 \text{ (Squares Counted)} \times 0.004 \; \mu l \text{ (Volume per Square)}} = 250,000 \text{ Cells}/\mu l$$

CORRECTIONS FOR CONTAMINATION

The specimen in the above example was obtained traumatically; therefore, a red blood cell count was performed so that a correlation for artificially introduced white cells could be calculated for the CSF white cell count. Red and white blood cell counts must also be performed on the patient's blood before it is possible to determine the number of white cells added by the peripheral blood contamination. By determining the ratio of WBCs to RBCs in the peripheral blood and comparing this ratio to the number of contaminating RBCs, the number of artificially added WBCs can be calculated using the formula:[21]

$$\text{WBC (added)} = \frac{\text{WBC (blood)} \times \text{RBC (CSF)}}{\text{RBC (blood)}}$$

A true CSF white blood cell count can then be obtained by subtracting the "added" WBCs from the actual count. When peripheral blood RBC and WBC counts are in the normal range, many laboratories choose to simply subtract either one or two cells for every 1200 RBCs or one cell for every 750 RBCs present in the CSF.[34] Studies have also shown that the actual WBC count is often lower than would be predicted from calculations using the peripheral blood WBC to RBC ratio. This indicates that some white cells must be lost, possibly at the bleeding site or during collection and transport.[30]

DIFFERENTIAL COUNT

Specimen Preparation

Once CSF has been found to contain cells, identifying the type or types of cells present is a valuable diagnostic aid. The differential count should be performed on a stained smear and not from the cells in the counting chamber. Poor visualization of the cells as they appear in the counting chamber has led to a common laboratory practice of reporting only the percentage of mononuclear and polynuclear cells present. To ensure that the maximum number of cells are available for examination, the specimen should be concentrated prior to the preparation of the smear. Methods available for specimen concentration include filtration, sedimentation, cytocentrifugation (Shandon Southern Instruments, Inc., Sewickey, Pennsylvania), and ordinary centrifugation. Most laboratories that do not have a cytocentrifuge concentrate specimens with ordinary centrifugation. The specimen is centrifuged for 5 to 10 minutes; supernatant fluid is removed and saved for additional tests; slides made from the suspended sediment are allowed to air-dry and are stained with Wright's stain. When performing the differential count, 100 cells should be counted, classified, and reported in terms of percentage. If the cell count is low and it is not possible to find 100 cells, report only the numbers of the cell types seen. An advantage to the filtration, sedimentation, and cytocentrifugation techniques is that they produce better cell yields. As little as 0.5 ml of CSF combined with dextran produces an adequate cell yield when processed with the cytocentrifuge.[31]

Significance of Normal Cells

The cells found in normal CSF are primarily lymphocytes and monocytes. Adults usually have a predominance of lymphocytes to monocytes (70:30); whereas monocytes are more prevalent in children.[22] Improved concentration methods are also showing occasional neutrophils in normal CSF.[20] The presence of increased numbers of these normal cells (termed pleocytosis) is considered abnormal, as is the finding of immature leukocytes, eosinophils, plasma cells, macrophages, increased tissue cells, and malignant cells. The CSF differential count is most frequently associated with its role in providing diagnostic information about the type of microorganism that is causing an infection of the meninges (meningitis). A high CSF white cell count of which the majority of the cells are neutrophils is considered indicative of bacterial meningitis. Likewise, a moderately elevated CSF white cell count with a high percentage of lymphocytes and monocytes suggests a meningitis of viral, tubercular, fungal, or parasitic origin. A low cell count, below 25 cells per cubic milliliter, with increased mononuclear cells is indicative of multiple sclerosis.[35] With this preliminary laboratory information and clinical observations, the physician can begin treatment without having to wait for the microbiology reports.

Significance of Abnormal Cells

As can be seen from Table 7-2, many pathologic conditions other than meningitis can be associated with the finding of abnormal cells in the CSF. Therefore, laboratory personnel should be careful not to overlook other types of cells because they become so accustomed to finding neutrophils, lymphocytes, and monocytes. The same care that is applied to reporting the blood differential should be given the CSF differential, keeping in mind that an even larger variety of cells is found in the CSF. Cell forms

TABLE 7-2. Predominant Cells Seen in Cerebrospinal Fluid

Type of Cell	Major Clinical Significance	Microscopic Findings
Lymphocyte	Normal Viral, tubercular, and fungal meningitis Multiple sclerosis	All stages of development may be found
Neutrophil	Bacterial meningitis Early cases of viral, tubercular, or fungal meningitis Cerebral hemorrhage	Granules may be less prominent than in blood[20] Cells disintegrate rapidly
Monocyte	Chronic bacterial meningitis Viral, tubercular, and fungal meningitis Multiple sclerosis	Found mixed with lymphocytes and neutrophils
Eosinophil	Parasitic infections Allergic reactions Intracranial shunts (hydrocephalus)	Same appearance as seen in blood
Macrophages	Viral and tubercular meningitis RBCs in spinal fluid	May contain phagocytized RBCs appearing as empty vacuoles or ghost cells and hemosiderin granules
Pia Arachnoid Mesothelial (PAM) Cells	Normal, mixed reactions, including neutrophils, lymphocytes, monocytes, and plasma cells	Resemble young monocytes with a round, not indented, nucleus[21]
Blast Forms	Acute leukemia	Lymphoblasts or myeloblasts
Plasma Cells	Multiple Sclerosis Lymphocyte reactions	Transitional and classic forms seen
Ependymal Cells Choroidal Cells	Normal trauma Diagnostic procedures	Seen in clusters with distinct nuclei and distinct cell walls
Malignant Cells	Metastatic carcinomas	Seen in clusters with fusing of cell borders and nuclei

differing from those found in blood include macrophages, choroid plexus and ependymal cells, and malignant cells. Macrophages appear within hours after the introduction of red blood cells into the fluid; therefore, the finding of increased macrophages containing red blood cells, which often appear as ghost cells or empty vacuoles, is indicative of a previous hemorrhage.[13] The macrophages may appear as giant cells and may also contain hemosiderin granules. Clusters of choroid plexus and ependymal cells from the lining of the ventricles are not considered clinically significant. They are most frequently seen following diagnostic procedures such as pneumoencephalography. Since many forms of malignant cells also appear in clusters, it is important to determine if the cells in a cluster are normal or abnormal. Normal cells will contain individually distinct cell walls and uniform nuclei; whereas malignant cells have a tendency toward irregularities of nuclei and fusing of cell walls. Malignant cells must be differentiated from similarly appearing benign meningeal cells. Any suspicious findings should be referred to the pathologist. (See color plates.)

CSF IN THE CHEMISTRY LABORATORY

Since CSF is formed by filtration of the plasma, one would expect to find the same chemicals in the CSF as are found in the plasma. This is essentially true; however, because the filtration process is selective and the chemical composition is also adjusted by the blood-brain barrier, normal values for CSF chemicals are not the same as the plasma values. Abnormal values are the result of alterations in the permeability of the blood-brain barrier or increased production or metabolism by the neural cells in response to a pathologic condition, and they seldom have the same diagnostic significance as plasma abnormalities. The clinically important CSF chemicals are relatively few in number, although under certain conditions, it may be necessary to measure a larger variety. We will concentrate on the most routinely requested analyses.

CSF PROTEIN

NORMAL PROTEIN COMPOSITION

The most frequently performed chemical test on CSF is the protein determination. Normal CSF contains a very small amount of protein. Normal values for total CSF protein are usually listed as 15 to 45 mg per dl, with slightly higher values found in infants and elderly people. Notice that this value is reported in milligrams per deciliter and not grams per deciliter, as are plasma protein concentrations. In general, the CSF contains protein fractions similar to those found in serum; however, as can be seen in Table 7-3, the ratio of CSF proteins to serum proteins varies among the fractions. As in serum, albumin comprises the majority of CSF protein. But in contrast to serum, prealbumin is the second most prevalent fraction in CSF. The alpha globulins include primarily haptoglobin and ceruloplasmin. Transferrin is the major beta globulin present, although a separate carbohydrate-deficient transferrin fraction, referred to as "tau," is seen in CSF and not in serum. CSF gamma globulin is primarily IgG, with only a small amount of IgA. IgM, fibrinogen, and beta lipoprotein are not found in normal CSF.[10]

CLINICAL SIGNIFICANCE OF ELEVATED PROTEIN

Elevated total protein values are most frequently seen in pathologic conditions, but abnormally low values will be present when fluid is leaking from the central nervous system. The causes of elevated CSF protein include damage to the blood-brain barrier, production of immunoglobulins within the central nervous system, decreased clearance of normal protein from the fluid, and degeneration of neural tissue. Meningitis and hemorrhage, conditions which result in damage to the blood-brain barrier, are the most common causes of elevated CSF protein. They, of course, are also associated with the production of cloudy fluids and increased cell counts. However, many other neurologic disorders can cause an elevation in the CSF protein, and it is not unusual to find an abnormal result on a clear fluid with a low cell count. Also, just as blood cells can be artificially introduced into a specimen by a traumatic tap, so can plasma protein. A

TABLE 7-3. CSF and Serum Protein Correlations*

	CSF (mg/dl)	Serum (mg/dl)	Ratio
Prealbumin	1.7	23.8	14
Albumin	15.5	3600	236
Ceruloplasmin	0.1	36.6	366
Transferrin	1.4	204	142
IgG	1.2	987	802
IgA	0.13	175	1346

*Adapted from Fishman.[10]

correction calculation similar to that used in cell counts is available for protein measurements; however, if the correction is to be used, it is essential that both the cell count and the protein determination be done on the same tube.[12] When the hematocrit and serum protein values are normal, it is acceptable to subtract 1 mg per dl protein for every 1200 RBCs counted.[21]

METHODOLOGY

The two most routinely used techniques for measuring total CSF protein utilize the principles of turbidity production or dye-binding ability. Turbidimetric methods have been available for many years and rely on the precipitation of protein by either sulfosalicylic acid or trichloroacetic acid. The reagent of choice is trichloroacetic acid because it will precipitate both albumin and globulin equally. Unless sulfosalicylic acid is combined with sodium sulfate, albumin will contribute more to the turbidity than globulin. Standards should be prepared from human serum and not from albumin. Dye-binding techniques offer the advantages of smaller sample size and less interference from external sources. The turbidimetric method using trichloroacetic acid has also been adapted to the Automated Chemistry Analyzer (ACA, Dupont Company, Wilmington, Delaware). The recent development of dye-binding procedures that are almost as rapid and easy to perform as the turbidity methods has greatly increased their acceptance in laboratories. A convenient laboratory procedure is provided by the Microprotein Rapid Stat Kit (Pierce Chemical Company, Rockford, Illinois). This method utilizes the dye Coomassie Brilliant Blue G-250 and the principle of "protein error of indicators" discussed in Chapter 4. Coomassie Brilliant Blue dye is used because it will bind to a variety of proteins rather than just to albumin. The color change of the pH-stabilized dye reagent from red to blue occurs when protein binds to the dye.[14] The concentration of protein present will determine the amount of blue color produced, thereby allowing a mathematical conversion of the intensity of the blue color present to the concentration of protein present (Beer's law).

Until recently, biuret used routinely for serum protein analysis had not been considered sensitive enough for CSF analysis. A modification of the biuret method that measures the rate of alkaline biuret–protein chelate formation rather than the colorimetric endpoint reaction has been incorporated by the Astra (Automated Stat/Routine Analyzer, Beckman Instruments Incorporated, Brea, California). The method can accurately determine CSF protein concentrations between 12 and 750 mg per dl and correlates well with measurements on the Automated Chemistry Analyzer.[9]

PROTEIN FRACTIONS

Both the turbidimetric and the dye-binding techniques are designed to measure total protein concentration. However, diagnosis of neurologic disorders associated with abnormal CSF protein often requires measurement of the individual protein fractions. Protein that appears in the CSF as a result of damage to the integrity of the blood-brain barrier will contain fractions proportional to those in plasma, with albumin present in the highest concentration. Diseases, including multiple sclerosis, that stimulate the immunocompetent cells in the central nervous system will show a higher proportion of IgG.[38] To determine if IgG is increased because it is being produced within the central nervous system or is only elevated owing to increased serum levels, an IgG profile is performed. The profile consists of an IgG to albumin ratio and an IgG index. Since albumin is not produced within the central nervous system, increased IgG accompanied by increased albumin represents damage to the barrier, and the ratio will resemble that of normal CSF. In contrast, production of IgG within the central nervous system will raise the IgG to albumin ratio. Because variations in the serum albumin concentrations can affect the IgG to albumin ratio, a more precise evaluation can be made using the IgG index.[16] The formula for this index is:[37]

$$\frac{\text{IgG/Albumin (CSF)}}{\text{IgG/Albumin (Serum)}}$$

By controlling for variations in serum albumin, actual synthesis of IgG within the central nervous system can be assessed. Conditions that do not involve central nervous system production of IgG have an index of less than 0.85; whereas a higher index is seen in multiple sclerosis.[5]

ELECTROPHORESIS

Electrophoresis performed on concentrated fluid is the method of choice for protein fractionation. The recommended support medium is agarose gel, and several commercial systems are available.[19] On agarose gel, a characteristic oligoclonal banding can be seen in up to 95 percent of patients with multiple sclerosis.[6] Oligoclonal bands can be seen in other diseases of immune origin; however, in the majority of these cases, oligoclonal bands are also found on serum electrophoresis and represent specific antibodies.[3] In multiple sclerosis, banding is not seen in serum, and the bands are characteristic for each patient rather than a specific antibody.[5] Immunofixation electrophoresis and isoelectric focusing techniques can also be used to detect oligoclonal banding and will demonstrate very small bands.[1]

Other procedures that are associated with the fractionation of CSF protein include serologic methods for the detection of myelin-based protein from the degradation of neural tissue, and two previously used tests, the Pandy and colloidal gold tests.

CSF GLUCOSE

Glucose enters the CSF by selective transport across the blood-brain barrier, which results in a normal value that is approximately 60 to 70 percent that of the plasma glucose. If the plasma glucose is 100 mg per dl, then a normal CSF glucose would be approximately 65 mg per dl. For an accurate evaluation of CSF glucose, it is necessary to run a blood glucose test for comparison. CSF glucose is analyzed using the same procedures employed for blood glucose. Specimens should be tested immediately because glycolysis occurs rapidly in the CSF. As will be seen shortly, a decreased value due to in vitro glycolysis could produce a serious error in patient treatment.

CLINICAL SIGNIFICANCE

The diagnostic significance of CSF glucose is confined to the finding of values that are decreased in relation to plasma values. Elevated CSF glucose is always a result of plasma elevations. Low CSF glucose values can be of considerable diagnostic value in determining the causative agents in meningitis. The finding of a markedly decreased CSF glucose accompanied by an increased white cell count and a large percentage of neutrophils is most indicative of bacterial meningitis. If the white cells are lymphocytes instead of neutrophils, tubercular meningitis is suspected. Likewise, if a normal CSF glucose is found with an increased number of lymphocytes, the diagnosis would favor viral meningitis. Keep in mind that classic laboratory patterns such as those just described may not be found in all cases of meningitis, but they can be helpful when they are present. Decreased CSF glucose values are thought to be caused primarily by alterations in the mechanisms of glucose transport across the blood-brain barrier, and to a smaller extent by increased utilization of glucose by the brain cells. Consumption of glucose by the microorganisms and leukocytes that are present in the fluid could not account for such decreased values, as it would not be possible to explain the variations in glucose concentrations seen in the different types of meningitis.[26]

CSF LACTATE

Although serum lactate levels are not routinely performed in the chemistry laboratory, the determination of CSF lactate levels is becoming a valuable aid in the diagnosis and management of meningitis cases. In bacterial, tubercular, and fungal meningitis, the elevation of CSF lactate to levels above 25 mg per dl occurs much more consistently than does the depression of glucose and provides the physician with more reliable information when the initial diagnosis is difficult.[2] CSF lactate levels remain elevated during initial treatment but fall rapidly when treatment is successful, thus offering a sensitive method for evaluating the effectiveness of antibiotic therapy.

Destruction of tissue within the central nervous system due to oxygen deprivation causes the production of increased CSF lactic acid levels. Therefore, elevated CSF lactate is not limited to meningitis and can result from any condition that decreases the flow of oxygen to the tissues.[33] However, the primary clinical significance at this time is in the diagnosis and treatment of meningitis.

CSF GLUTAMINE

Another chemical test that is frequently performed on CSF and not on blood is the glutamine test. Glutamine is produced in the central nervous system by the brain cells from ammonia and α-ketoglutarate. This process serves to remove the toxic metabolic waste product, ammonia, from the central nervous system. The normal concentration of glutamine in the CSF is 8 to 18 mg per dl.[17] Elevated levels are found in association with liver disorders that result in increased blood and CSF ammonia. Increased synthesis of glutamine is caused by the excess ammonia that is present in the central nervous system; therefore, the determination of CSF glutamine provides an indirect test for the presence of excess ammonia in the CSF. Several methods of assaying glutamine are available and are based on the measurement of ammonia liberated from the glutamine.[11] This is preferred over the direct measurement of CSF ammonia because the concentration of glutamine remains more stable than that of the volatile ammonia in the collected specimen.[10] The CSF glutamine level also correlates with clinical symptoms much better than does the blood ammonia.[17]

As the concentration of ammonia in the CSF increases, the supply of α-ketoglutarate becomes depleted; glutamine can no longer be produced to remove the toxic ammonia, and coma ensues. Some disturbance of consciousness is almost always seen when glutamine levels are over 35 mg per dl. Therefore, the CSF glutamine test is a recommended procedure for all patients with coma of unknown origin. Requests for the test also have increased recently because 75 percent of children with Reye's syndrome have elevated CSF glutamine.[11]

CSF LACTIC DEHYDROGENASE

Throughout the years, many enzymes in the CSF have been studied, but little clinical application of CSF enzyme tests has resulted. However, the development of techniques for separating and measuring the isoenzymes of lactic dehydrogenase has renewed interest in the CSF enzymes.[7] Lactic dehydrogenase can be separated into five isoenzymes, termed LD1, LD2, LD3, LD4, and LD5. The LD isoenzymes appear in the CSF following the destruction of particular cells, primarily neutrophils, lymphocytes, and brain cells. Brain tissue contains LD1 and LD2; lymphocytes contain LD2 and LD3; and neutrophils contain LD4 and LD5.[29] Therefore, LD isoenzymes can be utilized to confirm the presence of neutrophils and lymphocytes in the CSF, thereby aiding in the diagnosis of meningitis and, in cases of viral meningitis, providing an indication of the amount of tissue destruction that is occurring.

SUMMARY OF CSF CHEMISTRY TESTS

PROTEIN

1. Normal concentration is 15 to 45 mg per dl.
2. Elevated values are most frequently seen in meningitis, hemorrhage, and multiple sclerosis.

GLUCOSE

1. Normal value is 60 to 70 percent of the plasma concentration.
2. Decreased levels are seen with bacterial and tubercular meningitis.

LACTATE

1. Levels above 25 mg per dl are found with bacterial, tubercular, and fungal meningitis.

GLUTAMINE

1. Normal concentration is 8 to 18 mg per dl.
2. Levels above 35 mg per dl are associated with some disturbance of consciousness.

LACTIC DEHYDROGENASE

1. Isoenzymes LD1 and LD2 are found in brain tissue.
2. Isoenzymes LD2 and LD3 are found in lymphocytes.
3. Isoenzymes LD4 and LD5 are found in neutrophils.

CSF IN THE MICROBIOLOGY LABORATORY

The role of the microbiology laboratory in the analysis of CSF lies in the identification of the causative agent in cases of meningitis. For positive identification, the microorganism must be recovered from the fluid by growing it on the appropriate culture media. This can take anywhere from 24 hours in cases of bacterial meningitis to 6 weeks for tubercular meningitis. Consequently, in many instances, the CSF culture is actually a confirmatory rather than a diagnostic procedure. However, the microbiology laboratory does have several methods available to provide information so that a preliminary diagnosis can be made. These methods include the Gram stain, acid-fast stain, India ink preparation, Limulus Lysate test, counterimmunoelectrophoresis, and latex agglutination tests.

GRAM STAIN

The Gram stain is routinely performed on CSF from all suspected cases of meningitis, although its value lies in the detection of bacterial and fungal organisms. All smears and cultures should be performed on concentrated specimens because often only a few organisms are present at the onset of the disease. The CSF is normally centrifuged and slides and cultures prepared from the sediment. Even when concentrated specimens are used, there is at least a 10 percent chance that cultures will be negative. Thus, it is also recommended that blood cultures be taken since the causative organisms will often be present in both the CSF and the blood.[20] A CSF Gram stain is one of the most difficult slides to interpret because the number of organisms present is usually small and they can easily be overlooked, resulting in a false-negative report. Also, false-positive reports can occur if precipitated stain or debris is mistaken for microorganisms. Therefore, considerable care should be taken when interpreting a Gram stain.

Acid-fast or fluorescent antibody stains are not routinely performed on specimens, unless tubercular meningitis is suspected. Considering the length of time required to culture mycobacteria, a positive report from this smear is extremely valuable. Specimens from possible cases of fungal meningitis are Gram stained, but they should also have an India ink preparation performed on them. The India ink preparation is designed to detect one of the most common causes of fungal meningitis, *Cryptococcus neoformans.* However, it is not as sensitive as the reverse latex agglutination tests.[36]

LIMULUS LYSATE TEST

The Limulus Lysate test is relatively new to the field of CSF analysis; however, it is of great value in the diagnosis of meningitis caused by gram-negative bacteria.[27] The reagent for this test is prepared from the blood cells of the horseshoe crab (*Limulus polyphemus*). These cells, termed amebocytes, contain a copper complex that gives them a blue color, thereby making the horseshoe crab a true "blue blood." Endotoxin found in the cell walls of gram-negative bacteria coagulates the amebocyte lysate within 1 hour if incubated at 37°C. The test is sensitive to minute amounts of endotoxin and will detect all gram-negative bacteria. The procedure must be performed using sterile technique to prevent false-positive results due to contamination of specimens or tubes with endotoxin.

Counterimmunoelectrophoresis (CIE) is a serologic procedure utilized by the microbiology laboratory for detection and identification of bacterial antigens in the CSF. Although it is not as sensitive as the Limulus Lysate test, if positive, it provides rapid identification of the infectious organism.[8] Since not all bacteria possess the chemical characteristics needed for the reaction to take place, CIE is limited to the detection and identification of *Hemophilus influenzae, Streptococcus pneumoniae, Neisseria meningitidis, Escherichia coli,* and group B streptococci. Cross-over reactions, including one between *E. coli* and *H. influenzae,* may occur between these organisms.[8]

CSF IN THE SEROLOGY LABORATORY

Serologic examination of the CSF has historically been associated with the diagnosis of tertiary syphilis or neurosyphilis. The use of penicillin in the early stages of syphilis has greatly reduced the number of cases of neurosyphilis. Consequently, the number of requests for serologic tests for syphilis on CSF is lower. However, detection of the antibodies associated with syphilis in the CSF still remains a necessary diagnostic procedure. Although many different serologic tests for syphilis are available when testing blood, the recommended procedure for testing CSF is the VDRL (Venereal Disease Research Laboratories) using sensitized antigen and quantitation.[18] The FTA-ABS (fluorescent treponemal antibody absorption) test should not be used because contamination by even a minute amount of FTA-reactive blood may produce a positive CSF reaction.[4]

Serologic procedures for the rapid identification of the microorganisms present in cases of meningitis are also becoming a more routine part of the CSF examination (Table 7-4). As mentioned earlier, the CIE test is actually a serologic procedure that is

TABLE 7-4. Major Laboratory Results for the Differential Diagnosis of Meningitis

Bacterial	Viral	Tubercular	Fungal
Elevated WBC Count	Elevated WBC Count	Elevated WBC Count	Elevated WBC Count
Neutrophils Present	Lymphocytes Present	Lymphocytes and Monocytes Present	Lymphocytes and Monocytes Present
Marked Protein Elevation	Moderate Protein Elevation	Moderate to Marked Protein Elevation	Moderate to Marked Protein Elevation
Decreased Glucose	Normal Glucose	Decreased Glucose	Normal to Decreased Glucose
Elevated Lactate	Normal Lactate	Elevated Lactate	Elevated Lactate
Elevated LD4 and LD5	Elevated LD2 and LD3		
Positive Limulus Lysate with Gram-Negative Organisms		Pellicle Formation	Positive India Ink with *Cryptococcus neoformans*

useful for the identification of certain organisms. Also, antisera to an even larger number of organisms are available for performing reverse latex agglutination tests that are sensitive to 0.06 mg per ml.

TEACHING CSF ANALYSIS

Many of the problems that occur in the analysis of CSF are the result of inadequate training of the personnel performing the tests. This is understandable when one considers that not only is CSF difficult to collect, there is often very little fluid left for student practice after the required tests have been run.

Preparation of simulated fluids by adding blood cells to saline has met with limited success due to the instability of the cells in saline and the inability to perform routine chemical analyses for glucose and protein. More satisfactory results can be achieved using the recently published procedure described below, which provides the teaching laboratory with a specimen suitable for all types of cell analyses and glucose and protein determinations. The advantages of this simulated spinal fluid over others include: the absence of bicarbonate, which may cause bubbling with acidic diluting fluids; the absence of calcium, to prevent clot formation when blood is added; stability for 48 hours under refrigeration; no distortion of cellular morphology; and the presence of glucose and protein.[23]

SIMULATED SPINAL FLUID (SSF) PROCEDURE*
EQUIPMENT AND REAGENTS

1. Whole blood collected the same day in EDTA. The "ideal" blood specimen for preparing SSF has a white count around 10×10^9 per liter, a low platelet count, and a normal-appearing differential with at least 20 percent lymphocytes. Five to 7 ml of blood are needed to prepare 50 ml of SSF.
2. HBSS, Hanks' balanced salt solution ($10\times$), without phenol red, sodium bicarbonate, calcium or magnesium. (Grand Island Biological Company, Grand Island, New York) Dilute 1:10 with deionized water.
3. Thirty percent bovine serum albumin (BSA).
4. Macrohematocrit tubes.
5. Capillary (Pasteur type) pipettes—both standard and 9-inch length.
6. Horizontal head centrifuge. A Beckman TJ6 model (Beckman Instruments, Inc., Palo Alto, California) was used for this study.

PROCEDURE

1. For each SSF sample, dispense 50 ml diluted balanced salt solution into a 125-ml Erlenmeyer flask. (The amount of balanced salt solution may be varied; 50 ml will make approximately 30 aliquots of SSF.)
2. Centrifuge the blood in the original collection tube at $300 \times g$ for 5 minutes. A gray-pink buffy coat layer should be visible at the interface between the plasma and the red cells.
3. Aspirate off as much plasma as possible with a capillary pipette. Do not disturb the top (buffy coat) layer. Discard the plasma.
4. With a 9-inch capillary pipette and a circular motion, aspirate off the remaining plasma and the *entire* buffy coat layer. A small amount of the red cell layer will be aspirated into the pipette at the same time. This is acceptable.
5. Fill a macrohematocrit tube with this buffy coat mixture. Do not mix blood specimens from more than one source in one tube (they may agglutinate).

*From Lofsness and Jensen,[23] with permission.

6. Centrifuge the macrohematocrit tube at 900 × g for 10 minutes.
7. Pipette off as much of the plasma as possible and discard it. If a definite white layer (platelets) is visible above the gray buffy coat, carefully remove as much of it as possible without disturbing the gray layer.
8. Using a clean 9-inch capillary pipette, aspirate off the buffy coat (and as little of the red cell layer as possible) and add it to the flask containing diluted balanced salt solution. Rinse the pipette several times.
9. Mix well, and check the concentration of red cells and white cells by examining the SSF in a hemocytometer.
10. Adjust the concentration of cells as needed: add more balanced salt solution to decrease the number of red cells and white cells. The number of red cells may be increased by adding more cells from the red cell layer. Since the entire buffy coat has been utilized, it is not possible to increase the number of white cells.
11. Add one drop (approximately 0.05 ml) of 30 percent bovine serum albumin to each 50 ml of SSF for each 30 mg per dl total protein desired.
12. Mix well, and dispense aliquots of approximately 1.5 ml SSF into appropriate tightly stoppered containers.

REFERENCES

1. CAWLEY, LP, ET AL: *Immunofixation electrophoretic techniques applied to identification of proteins in serum and cerebrospinal fluid.* Clin Chem 22(8):1262–1268, 1976.
2. CONTRONI, G, ET AL: *Cerebrospinal fluid lactic acid levels in meningitis.* J Pediatr 91(3):379–384, 1977.
3. CUTLER, RWP AND SPERTELL, RB: *Cerebrospinal fluid: A selective review.* Ann Neurol 11(1):1–8, 1982.
4. DAVIS, LE AND SPERRY, S: *The CSF-FTA test and the significance of blood contamination.* Ann Neurol 6(1):68, 1979.
5. DELBECH, B AND LICHTBLAU, E: *Immunochemical estimation of IgG and albumin in cerebrospinal fluid.* Clin Chim Acta 37:15–23, 1972.
6. DELMOTTE, P AND CARTON, H: *Electrophoresis of cerebrospinal fluid proteins.* Clin Neurol Neurosurg 83(4):183, 1981.
7. DIGIORGIO, D: *Determination of serum lactic dehydrogenase isoenzymes by use of the Diagnostest cellulose acetate electrophoresis system.* Clin Chem 17:326–331, 1971.
8. FELDMAN, WE: *Relation of concentrations of bacteria and bacterial antigen in cerebrospinal fluid to prognosis in patients with bacterial meningitis.* N Engl J Med 296(8):433–435, 1977.
9. FINLEY, P AND WILLIAMS, J: *Assay of cerebrospinal fluid protein: A rate biuret method evaluation.* Clin Chem 29(1):126–129, 1983.
10. FISHMAN, RA: *Cerebrospinal Fluid in Diseases of the Nervous System.* WB Saunders, Philadelphia, 1980.
11. GLASGOW, AM AND DHIENSIRI, K: *Improved assay for spinal fluid glutamine and values for children with Reye's syndrome.* Clin Chem 20(6):642–644, 1974.
12. GLASSER, L: *Tapping the wealth of information in CSF.* Diagnostic Medicine 4(1):23–33, 1981.
13. GLASSER, L: *Cells in cerebrospinal fluid.* Diagnostic Medicine, 4(2):33–50, 1981.
14. GODD, K: *Protein estimation in spinal fluid using Coomassie Blue reagent.* Med Lab Sci 38:61–63, 1981.
15. HAMMOCK, M AND MILHORAT, T: *The cerebrospinal fluid: Current concepts of its formation.* Ann Clin Lab Sci 6(1):22–28, 1976.
16. HERSHEY, LA AND TROTTER, JL: *The use and abuse of the cerebrospinal fluid IgG profile in the adult: A practical evaluation.* Ann Neurol 8(4):426–434, 1980.

17. HOURANI, BT, HAMLIN, EM, AND REYNOLDS, TB: *Cerebrospinal fluid glutamine as a measure of hepatic encephalopathy.* Arch Intern Med 127:1033–1036, 1971.

18. JAFFE, HW: *The laboratory diagnosis of syphilis: New concepts.* Ann Intern Med 83(6):846–850, 1975.

19. JOHNSON, KP, ET AL: *Agarose electrophoresis of cerebrospinal fluid in multiple sclerosis.* Neurology 27:273–277, 1977.

20. KJELDSBERG, CR AND KNIGHT, JA: *Body Fluids, Laboratory Examination of Cerebrospinal, Synovial and Serous Fluids: A Textbook Atlas.* American Society of Clinical Pathologists, Chicago, 1982.

21. KJELDSBERG, CR AND KRIEG, A: *Cerebrospinal fluid and other body fluids.* In HENRY, JB (ED): *Clinical Diagnosis and Management by Laboratory Methods.* WB Saunders, Philadelphia, 1979.

22. KOLMEL, HW: *Atlas of Cerebrospinal Fluid Cells.* Springer-Verlag, New York, 1976.

23. LOFSNESS, KG AND JENSEN, TL: *The preparation of simulated spinal fluid for teaching purposes.* Am J Med Technol 49(7):493–496, 1983.

24. MATTHEWS, W AND FROMMEYER, W: *The in vitro behavior of erythrocytes in human cerebrospinal fluid.* J Lab Clin Med 45:508–515, 1955.

25. McCOMB, JG: *Recent research into the nature of cerebrospinal fluid formation and absorption.* J Neurosurg 59:369–383, 1983.

26. MENKES, J: *The causes of low spinal fluid sugar in bacterial meningitis: Another look.* Pediatrics 44(1):1–3, 1969.

27. NACHUM, R AND NEELY, M: *Clinical diagnostic usefulness of the Limulus Amoebocyte Lysate assay.* Laboratory Medicine 13(2):112–117, 1982.

28. NAGDA, KK: *Procoagulant activity of cerebrospinal fluid in health and disease.* Indian J Med Res 74:107–110, 1981.

29. NELSON, PV, CAREY, WF, AND POLLARD, AC: *Diagnostic significance and source of lactate dehydrogenase and its isoenzymes in cerebrospinal fluid of children with a variety of neurological disorders.* J Clin Pathol 28(10):828–833, 1975.

30. OSBORNE, J AND PIZER, B: *Effect on the white cell count of contaminating cerebrospinal fluid with blood.* Arch Dis Child 56(5):400–401, 1981.

31. PELC, S: *Cytocentrifugation of cerebrospinal fluid with dextran.* Acta Cytol 26:721–724, 1982.

32. PLUM, F AND SIESJO, B: *Recent advances in CSF physiology.* Anesthesiology 42(6):708–729, 1975.

33. PRYCE, JD, GANT, PW, AND SAUL, KJ: *Normal concentrations of lactate, glucose and protein in cerebrospinal fluid, and the diagnostic implications of abnormal concentrations.* Clin Chem 16(7):562–565, 1970.

34. RESKE, A, HAFERKAMP, G, AND HOPF, H: *Influence of artificial blood contamination on the analysis of cerebrospinal fluid.* J Neurol 226:187–193, 1981.

35. REUNANEN, MI: *Spontaneous proliferation of cerebrospinal fluid mononuclear cells in multiple sclerosis.* Journal of Neuroimmunology 3:275–283, 1982.

36. SALOM, I: *Cryptococcal meningitis: Significance of positive antigen test on undiluted spinal fluid.* NY State J Med 81(9):1369–1370, 1981.

37. TIBBLING, G, LINK, H, AND OHMAN, S: *Principles of albumin and IgG analyses in neurological disorders.* Scand J Clin Lab Invest 37:385–401, 1977.

38. TOURTELLOTTE, WW: *Cerebrospinal fluid in multiple sclerosis.* In VINKEN, PJ AND BRUYN, GW (EDS): *Handbook of Clinical Neurology.* Elsevier, New York, 1970.

STUDY QUESTIONS (Choose one best answer)

1. The functions of the cerebrospinal fluid include all of the following except:

   a. nutritional enrichment of nervous tissue
   b. transmittance of neurologic impulses
   c. removal of metabolic waste products
   d. protection of neurologic tissue from trauma

2. Three tubes of CSF labeled 1, 2, and 3 are received in the laboratory. They should be distributed as follows:

   a. hematology #1, chemistry #2, and microbiology #3
   b. hematology #2, chemistry #3, and microbiology #1
   c. hematology #3, chemistry #1, and microbiology #2
   d. hematology #1, chemistry #3, and microbiology #2

3. A xanthochromic CSF specimen will appear:

   a. crystal clear
   b. white and turbid
   c. yellow and clear
   d. red and turbid

4. Place the appropriate letter in front of the statement that best describes CSF specimens in these two conditions:

   a. Intracranial hemorrhage
   b. Traumatic tap
   ____ even distribution of blood in all three tubes
   ____ xanthochromic supernatant
   ____ concentration of blood in Tube 1 is greater than in Tube 3
   ____ specimen contains clots

5. White blood cell counts on clear CSF specimens are performed:

   a. using electronic counters
   b. only if more than 200 cells are present
   c. on undiluted specimens if there is no cell overlapping
   d. on specimens diluted 1:200 with gentian violet

6. Using a Neubauer counting chamber, 150 white blood cells are counted in an undiluted CSF specimen. Calculate the WBC count.

7. To determine the WBC count on a cloudy CSF specimen that contains both red and white blood cells, it is necessary to:

   a. dilute the specimen using glacial acetic acid containing gentian violet
   b. dilute the specimen using saline and gentian violet
   c. determine the percentage of polynuclear and mononuclear cells in the counting chamber
   d. centrifuge the specimen prior to diluting with saline and gentian violet

8. Calculate the WBCs per microliter on a CSF specimen diluted 1:20 when 60 cells are counted in the four large squares of a Neubauer chamber.

9. White blood cell counts on CSF specimens collected during a traumatic tap:

   a. should only be performed using electronic cell counters
   b. should not be performed from tubes containing streaks of blood
   c. should be corrected for white blood cells added by the traumatic tap
   d. should be corrected for both red and white blood cells added by the traumatic tap

10. Differential counts on CSF are performed on:

    a. cells as they are counted in the hemocytometer
    b. coverslipped wet preparations
    c. stained smears prepared from the undiluted specimen
    d. stained smears prepared from concentrated specimens

11. In meningitis, the CSF may contain increased numbers of all of the following cells except:

    a. lymphocytes
    b. ependymal
    c. monocytes
    d. neutrophils

12. Vacuolated macrophages are seen in the CSF following:

    a. cerebral hemorrhage
    b. traumatic tap
    c. allergic reactions
    d. pneumoencephalography

13. Clusters of choroidal and ependymal cells are seen in the CSF in:

    a. multiple sclerosis
    b. precancerous syndromes
    c. post-pneumoencephalography
    d. intracranial shunts

14. Chemical analysis of CSF shows that the fluid contains:

    a. plasma chemicals in the same concentration as in the plasma
    b. plasma chemicals in different concentrations than in the plasma
    c. more chemicals than are found in plasma
    d. fewer chemicals than are found in plasma

15. The normal CSF protein is:

    a. 15 to 45 mg/dl
    b. 15 to 45 g/dl
    c. 50 to 100 mg/dl
    d. 50 to 100 g/dl

16. Normal CSF protein differs from serum protein by the:

    a. presence of IgG
    b. presence of haptoglobin
    c. presence of ceruloplasmin
    d. absence of fibrinogen

17. Conditions that produce elevated CSF protein include all of the following except:

    a. fluid leakage
    b. meningitis
    c. multiple sclerosis
    d. hemorrhage

18. CSF protein measurements obtained using a turbidity method will not equally represent both albumin and globulin if:

    a. trichloroacetic acid is used
    b. sulfosalicylic acid is combined with sodium sulfate
    c. standards are made from human serum
    d. standards are made from human albumin

19. The Coomassie Blue dye-binding method for measuring CSF protein is based on the principle of:

    a. protein-dye precipitation
    b. protein error of indicators
    c. peptide bond and dye combination
    d. protein interference with dye binding to specific substrates

20. The IgG index is used to:

    a. confirm elevated CSF protein results
    b. detect increased levels of CSF IgG due to damage to the blood-brain barrier
    c. detect increased levels of CSF IgG due to production within the central nervous system
    d. detect increased levels of serum IgG that influence the CSF concentration

21. CSF electrophoresis to confirm the diagnosis of multiple sclerosis would be expected to show:

    a. increased IgG with oligoclonal bands not seen on serum electrophoresis
    b. increased IgG with oligoclonal bands similar to those seen on serum electrophoresis
    c. decreased IgG with antibody-specific oligoclonal bands
    d. decreased IgG with antibody-specific oligoclonal bands resembling those seen on serum electrophoresis

22. The normal CSF glucose is:

    a. 60 to 70 mg/dl
    b. 80 to 120 mg/dl
    c. 60 to 70 percent of the blood glucose
    d. 10 to 20 percent higher than the blood glucose

23. The primary cause of decreased CSF glucose in bacterial meningitis is:

    a. utilization of glucose by the microorganisms present in the fluid
    b. rapid glycolysis
    c. utilization of glucose by leukocytes present in the fluid
    d. alteration of blood-brain glucose transport

24. Measurement of CSF lactate levels is valuable for all of the following except:

    a. preliminary diagnosis of tubercular meningitis
    b. preliminary diagnosis of fungal meningitis
    c. monitoring the effects of antibiotic treatment
    d. distinguishing between tubercular and fungal meningitis

25. A major CSF chemical that is measured in suspected cases of Reye's syndrome is:

   a. glucose
   b. glutamine
   c. lactate
   d. lactic dehydrogenase

26. Lactic dehydrogenase isoenzymes appearing in the CSF are derived from:

   a. damage to the blood-brain barrier
   b. contamination due to traumatic tap
   c. neutrophils and lymphocytes
   d. neutrophils, lymphocytes, and brain cells

27. Gram stains performed on CSF specimens are of value in the:

   a. diagnosis of tubercular meningitis
   b. diagnosis of bacterial meningitis
   c. detection of viral meningitis
   d. detection of bacterial and fungal meningitis

28. Specimens from patients suspected of having fungal meningitis should be tested with:

   a. Gram stain, acid-fast stain, and India ink
   b. Gram stain and India ink
   c. India ink only
   d. acid-fast stain and India ink

29. The Limulus Lysate test will detect the presence of:

   a. gram-positive bacteria
   b. gram-negative bacteria
   c. acid-fast organisms
   d. all microorganisms

30. The serologic test for syphilis used for testing CSF is the:

   a. VDRL
   b. RPR
   c. FTA-ABS
   d. TPI

CASE STUDIES

1. Mary Howard, age 5, is admitted to the pediatrics ward with a temperature of 105°F, lethargy, and cervical rigidity. A lumbar spinal tap is performed, and three tubes of cloudy CSF are delivered to the laboratory. Preliminary test results are:

   WBC count: 4000 cells/mm^3
   Differential: 90% neutrophils, 10% lymphocytes
   Glucose: 10 mg/dl
   Protein: 150 mg/dl
   Gram stain: no organisms seen

a. From these results, what preliminary diagnosis could the physician consider?

b. Would any other tests be of value in the management of this patient?

c. Is the Gram stain result of particular significance?

2. A clear CSF specimen from a 35-year-old patient experiencing mild motor difficulties has a white blood cell count of 22 mononuclear cells/mm^3 and a total protein of 60 mg/dl.

a. Are these results of any significance?

b. If so, what additional tests might the physician order on this specimen?

c. What is a possible diagnosis for this patient?

3. Examination of the CSF from a 50-year-old woman suspected of having meningitis reveals a moderately elevated white blood cell count consisting primarily of mononuclear cells. The physician must make a preliminary diagnosis of viral, tubercular, or fungal meningitis.

a. Name the test that would provide the most valuable information in the diagnosis of each meningitis type, and explain its differential value.

b. What other tests would be of value in the differentiation of each type?

8
MISCELLANEOUS BODY FLUIDS

INSTRUCTIONAL OBJECTIVES

Upon completion of this chapter, readers will be able to:

1. discuss the composition of seminal fluid

2. instruct a patient in the correct method for collecting a semen specimen

3. list the normal values for semen volume, viscosity, pH, sperm count, motility, and morphology

4. calculate a sperm count when provided with the number of sperm counted, the dilution, and the area of the counting chamber used

5. describe the method used to evaluate sperm motility

6. list three tests used to evaluate infertility that are not part of the routine semen analysis

7. list two methods for identifying a questionable fluid as semen

8. discuss the composition and appearance of normal synovial fluid

9. list the five classifications of joint disorders, their pathologic significance, and the abnormal laboratory values associated with them

10. distinguish between a hemorrhagic arthritis and a traumatic aspiration

11. discuss the Ropes test, including methodology, grading, and significance

12. name four abnormal cells found in synovial fluid

13. discuss the principles of polarized and compensated polarized light and their significance in differentiating between monosodium urate and calcium pyrophosphate crystals

14. list four genera of bacteria frequently found in synovial fluid

15. define serous fluids

16. differentiate between transudates and exudates, including etiology, appearance, specific gravity, protein, and lactic dehydrogenase values

17. describe the appearance of normal pleural, pericardial, and peritoneal fluids

18. differentiate between a hemothorax and a hemorrhagic effusion

19. list three common chemical tests performed on pleural fluid and state their significance

20. state the purpose for performing a peritoneal lavage

21. list three common chemical tests performed on ascitic fluid and state their significance

22. discuss the physiology and composition of amniotic fluid

23. explain the principle and significance of the amniotic fluid bilirubin test

24. discuss the relationship of the lecithin-sphingomyelin ratio, shake test, phosphatidylglycerol, and amniotic fluid creatinine to fetal maturity

25. discuss the methodology of the sweat electrolyte test using pilocarpine iontophoresis and its role in the diagnosis of cystic fibrosis

This chapter includes sections on seminal fluid, synovial fluid, pleural, pericardial, and peritoneal fluids, amniotic fluid, and a brief discussion of sweat analysis. Although blood, urine, and cerebrospinal fluid are the most common specimens received in the clinical laboratory, one must also be prepared to analyze a variety of other fluids that are formed throughout the body. These fluids are often associated with specific conditions or diseases and may require specialized tests in addition to the examinations routinely performed on all specimens. Also, unlike urine and blood, these fluids are not easily collected or always available in large amounts, so utmost care must be taken to ensure that as much information as possible is obtained from the specimen. This is best accomplished by providing laboratory personnel with a thorough understanding of these fluids, including their compositions, routine and specialized test procedures, associated pathologies, and any unique precautions that must be taken.

SEMINAL FLUID

Of the fluids to be discussed in this chapter, seminal fluid is the specimen that is most frequently received in clinical laboratories. The two primary reasons for analysis are the evaluations of infertility cases and post-vasectomy patients. Identification of a fluid as semen can also be useful in forensic medicine.

Seminal fluid is composed of four fractions that are contributed individually by the bulbourethral and urethral glands, the testis and epididymis, the prostate, and the seminal vesicles (Fig. 8-1). Each fraction differs in its composition, and the mixing of all four fractions during ejaculation is necessary for the production of a normal semen specimen. Spermatozoa are produced in the testis and mature in the epididymis. They account for only a small amount of the total semen volume, the majority of which is supplied by the seminal vesicles in the form of a viscous liquid that furnishes fructose and other nutrients to maintain the spermatozoa. The other significant contribution is made by the prostate and consists of a milky fluid that contains acid phosphatase and proteolytic enzymes that act on the fluid from the seminal vesicles, resulting in the coagulation and liquefaction of the semen.[5]

The variety of the composition of the semen fractions makes proper collection of a complete specimen essential for accurate evaluation of male fertility. Patients should receive detailed instructions concerning specimen collection. Specimens should be collected in sterile containers following a 3-day period of sexual abstinence. The use of condoms for specimen collection is not recommended for fertility testing because the condoms may contain spermicidal agents. Post-vasectomy specimens, where only the presence of sperm, whether viable or nonviable, is significant, are not affected by condoms. Whenever possible, the specimen should be collected in a room provided by the laboratory. However, if this is not appropriate, the specimen should be kept at room temperature and delivered to the laboratory within 1 hour. The time of specimen collection, not specimen receipt, must be recorded by the laboratory. A fresh semen

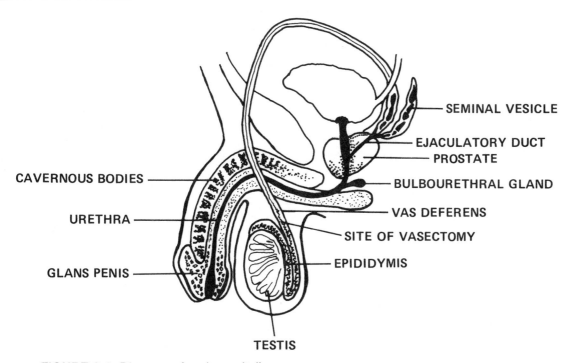

CAVERNOUS BODIES

URETHRA

GLANS PENIS

SEMINAL VESICLE

EJACULATORY DUCT

PROSTATE

BULBOURETHRAL GLAND

VAS DEFERENS

SITE OF VASECTOMY

EPIDIDYMIS

TESTIS

FIGURE 8-1. Diagram of male genitalia.

specimen is clotted and should liquify within 30 minutes after collection; therefore, the time of collection is essential for evaluation of semen liquefaction. Analysis of the specimen cannot begin until after liquefaction has occurred.

When evaluating semen specimens in cases of infertility, the following parameters are routinely measured: volume, viscosity, pH, sperm count, motility, and morphology. Normal values are shown in Table 8-1.

VOLUME AND VISCOSITY

Normal semen volume ranges between 2 and 5 ml and is measured by pouring the specimen into a graduated cylinder. Viscosity can be determined as the specimen is being poured into the cylinder. A specimen of normal viscosity will pour in droplets and will not appear clumped or stringy. Always be sure that the specimen has completely liquified prior to determining viscosity. Increased viscosity or incomplete liquefaction will interfere with sperm motility. Any abnormal appearance of the fluid, such as the presence of blood, pigmentation, or increased turbidity, that may be due to white blood cells should also be noted at this time.

TABLE 8-1. Normal Values for Semen Analysis

Volume	2–5 ml
Viscosity	Pours in droplets
pH	7.3–7.8
Count	40–160 million/ml
Motility	>50–60% within 3 hours Quality >2.0 or fair
Morphology	<30% Abnormal forms

pH

The pH of normal semen is slightly alkaline, with a range of 7.3 to 7.8, and can be measured using pH testing paper.[23] An abnormally high ratio of prostatic fluid to seminal fluid will produce a more acidic pH.

SPERM COUNT

Even though fertilization is accomplished by one spermatozoa, the actual number of sperm present in a semen specimen is a valid measurement of fertility. Normal values are commonly listed as 40 to 160 million sperm per milliliter, with counts between 20 and 40 million per milliliter considered borderline. The sperm count is performed in the same manner as the blood and CSF counts, that is, by diluting the specimen and counting the cells in a Neubauer chamber. The amount of the dilution and the number of squares counted vary among laboratories. Two frequently used methods dilute the specimen 1:20 using a Thoma white blood cell pipette and count the sperm in either the five RBC squares or in two large WBC squares (see Fig. 7-4). When the five RBC squares are used, the number of sperm counted is multiplied by 1,000,000 to calculate the number of sperm per milliliter.[23,38] If the two WBC squares are used, the count is multiplied by 100,000 to achieve the same result.[5]

The basic cell counting formula discussed in Chapter 7 can also be applied to sperm counts. But since this formula provides the number of cells per microliter, the figure must then be multiplied by 1000 to give the number of sperm per milliliter.

Example: 1. Using a 1:20 dilution, 600 sperm are counted in the two WBC counting squares. Calculate the sperm count per milliliter.

A. 600 Sperm Counted $\times$ 100,000 = 60,000,000 Sperm/ml

B. $$\frac{600 \text{ Sperm} \times 20 \text{ (Dilution)}}{2 \text{ (Squares Counted)} \times 0.1 \text{ } \mu l \text{ (Volume Counted)}}$$

= 60,000,000 Sperm/μl

60,000 Sperm/μl $\times$ 1,000 = 60,000,000 Sperm/ml

2. Using a 1:20 dilution, 60 sperm are counted in the five RBC counting squares. Calculate the sperm count per milliliter.

A. 60 Sperm Counted $\times$ 1,000,000 = 60,000,000 Sperm/ml

B. $$\frac{60 \text{ Sperm} \times 20 \text{ (Dilution)}}{5 \text{ (Squares Counted)} \times 0.004 \text{ } \mu l \text{ (Volume Counted)}}$$

= 60,000 Sperm/μl

60,000 Sperm/μl $\times$ 1,000 = 60,000,000 Sperm/ml

Dilution of the semen prior to counting is essential to provide for immobilization of the sperm. The traditional diluting fluid contains sodium bicarbonate and formalin, which immobilize and preserve the cells; however, good results can also be achieved using tap water.[23] Care should be taken not to contaminate the specimen with diluting fluid prior to determining the motility. Both dilutions and counts should be performed in duplicate on completely liquified specimens to ensure accuracy.

MOTILITY

Equal to, if not more important than, the number of sperm present is the motility of the sperm, because once presented to the cervix, the sperm must propel themselves through the fallopian tubes to the ovum. Laboratory evaluation of sperm motility is a subjective procedure that is performed by examining the undiluted specimen microscopically and determining the percentage of sperm showing active motility. Sperm should be evaluated on their progressive forward movement, and any motility due to brownian movement should be disregarded. Many laboratories not only report the percentage of motile sperm, but also grade the motility either on a scale of 0 to 4, with 4 indicating rapid progressive movement, or by word descriptions ranging from poor to excellent. Approximately 25 high-power fields should be examined. The percentage and quality of motility should be determined in each field, and an average of these results should be reported. Various time frames have been established for the determination of motility, with some laboratories testing the specimen at periodic intervals up to 24 hours. However, the common practice is to observe motility within 3 hours of collection but not before liquefaction has taken place. A minimum motility of 50 to 60 percent with a quality of fair (2.0) is considered normal for specimens tested within the 3-hour time period.[5]

MORPHOLOGY

Just as the presence of a normal number of sperm that are nonmotile will produce infertility, the presence of sperm that are morphologically incapable of fertilization will also result in infertility. Sperm morphology is evaluated with respect to both head and tail appearance. The normal sperm has an oval head measuring approximately 3×5 μm and a long, tapering tail. Abnormalities in head structure (Fig. 8-2) are associated with poor ovum penetration and include double heads, giant and amorphous heads, pinheads, tapering heads, and constricted heads. Motility is impeded in sperm with double or coiled tails. Immature sperm (spermatids) may also be present and must be differentiated from white blood cells. They are more spherical than mature sperm and may or may not have tails. The presence of a high number of immature forms is considered abnormal because sperm usually mature within the epididymis prior to their release. Sperm morphology should be reported from a stained specimen examined under oil immersion. The recommended stain is the Papanicolaou. However, if this is not available, acceptable results can be obtained using hematoxylin, crystal violet, or Giemsa stains.[13] At least 200 spermatozoa should be examined and the percentage of abnormal forms reported. A specimen that contains less than 30 percent abnormal forms is considered normal.

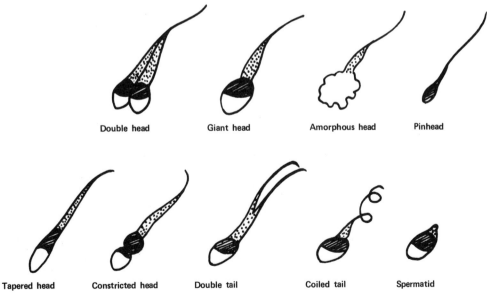

| Double head | Giant head | Amorphous head | Pinhead |

| Tapered head | Constricted head | Double tail | Coiled tail | Spermatid |

FIGURE 8-2. Abnormal sperm morphology.

TABLE 8-2. Additional Testing for Abnormal Semen Analysis

Abnormal Result	Possible Abnormality	Test
Decreased motility with normal count	Viability	Eosin-nigrosin stain
Decreased count	Lack of seminal vesicle support medium	Fructose level
Decreased motility with clumping	Male anti-sperm antibodies	Sperm agglutination with male plasma
Normal analysis with continued infertility	Female anti-sperm antibodies	Sperm agglutination with female plasma

Should abnormalities be discovered in any of these routine parameters, additional tests may be requested (Table 8-2). The most common are tests for sperm viability, seminal fluid fructose level, and sperm agglutinins. Concern about the viability of sperm arises when a specimen has a normal count and markedly decreased motility. Viability is tested by mixing the specimen with an eosin-nigrosin stain and examining microscopically for dead cells that stain red against a purple background. Living cells are not infiltrated by the eosin dye and remain a bluish white color. Low sperm counts may be caused by a lack of support medium produced in the seminal vesicles, which is indicated by a low to absent fructose level in the semen specimen. Sperm agglutinating antibodies may be present in the plasma of either the male or his female partner and will result in the clumping and inactivation of the sperm. The presence of antibodies in the male plasma can be suspected when clumps of sperm are observed during a routine semen analysis; whereas the presence of anti-sperm antibodies in the female will result in a normal semen analysis accompanied by continued infertility. Confirmation of sperm agglutinating antibodies is accomplished by mixing the semen specimen with the appropriate male or female serum and observing the agglutination or immobilization of the sperm.[13] Quantitation of anti-spermatozoa antibodies can be performed with solid-phase radioimmunoassay using ^{125}I bacterial protein-A.[8]

Post-vasectomy semen analysis is a much less involved procedure when compared to the infertility analysis, since the only concern is the presence or absence of spermatozoa. The length of time required for complete sterilization to occur can vary greatly among patients and depends on both time and number of ejaculations. Therefore, it is not uncommon to find viable sperm in a post-vasectomy patient, and care should be taken not to overlook even a single sperm. Specimens are routinely tested at monthly intervals beginning at two months post-vasectomy and continuing until two consecutive monthly specimens show no spermatozoa. Recommended testing includes microscopic examination of samples from both the mixed undiluted specimen and the sediment from the centrifuged specimen.[38]

On certain occasions, the laboratory may be called upon to determine if semen is actually present in a specimen. A primary example of this is in cases of alleged rape. It may be possible to microscopically examine the specimen for the presence of sperm; however, a more reliable procedure is to chemically test the material for acid phosphatase content. Because seminal fluid is the only body fluid with a high concentration of acid phosphatase, the detection of this enzyme can confirm the presence of semen in a specimen. Further information can often be obtained by performing ABO blood grouping and HLA testing on the specimen.

SYNOVIAL FLUID

Synovial fluid, often referred to as "joint fluid," is a viscous liquid found in the joint cavities (Fig. 8-3). It is formed as an ultrafiltrate of the plasma across the synovial

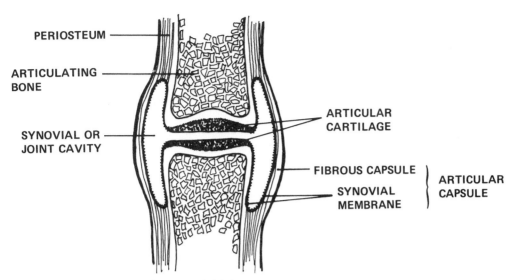

FIGURE 8-3. Diagram of a synovial joint.

membrane, into which a mucopolysaccharide containing hyaluronic acid and a small amount of protein is secreted by the cells of the synovial membrane. Except for the high molecular weight proteins, the plasma filtration is nonselective; therefore, normal synovial fluid has essentially the same chemical composition as the plasma. Synovial fluid supplies nutrients to the cartilage and acts as a lubricant to the surfaces of the frequently moving joints.

COLLECTION

Although the fluid is found in all joints, the specimen usually received in the laboratory is an aspirate of the knee. Synovial fluid is collected by needle aspiration, called arthrocentesis. The normal amount of fluid contained in the knee cavity is less than 3.5 ml; however, this amount increases in disorders of the joints.[14] Therefore, the volume of fluid collected is dependent on the degree of fluid buildup in the joints. Normal synovial fluid will not clot; however, fluid from a diseased joint may contain fibrinogen and form a clot. Therefore, both anticoagulated and nonanticoagulated specimens should be collected. Recommended specimen containers include:[34]

1. EDTA (sequestrin) tube for cell counts and differentials. When using commercially prepared EDTA tubes, the specified amount of fluid should be added because artifacts may occur if too little fluid is mixed with the anticoagulant.
2. Heparinized tube for chemical and immunologic tests. Specimens should be centrifuged and the fluid separated from the cells as soon as possible to prevent the addition of intracellular constituents to the fluid. Fluid for complement studies should be frozen before storage.
3. Plain, sterile tube for microbiologic testing and crystal examination.

Analysis of synovial fluid is used to classify joint disorders in terms of their pathologic origins.[35] The five commonly used categories associated with fluid buildup and arthritis, and their clinical significance, are listed in Table 8-3. Results from both synovial fluid and blood analyses must be considered along with the patient's clinical history before a category is assigned (Table 8-4).

SYNOVIAL FLUID IN THE HEMATOLOGY LABORATORY

The major portion of the routine synovial fluid analysis takes place in the hematology laboratory and includes a report of the appearance, viscosity, cell count, cell differential, and crystal identification. Normal synovial fluid appears clear and pale yellow. The color

TABLE 8-3. Classification and Pathologic Significance of Joint Disorders[35]

Group Classification	Pathologic Significance
I. Noninflammatory	Degenerative joint disorders
II. Inflammatory	Immunologic problems, including rheumatoid arthritis and lupus erythematosus
III. Septic	Microbial infection
IV. Crystal-Induced	Gout Pseudogout
V. Hemorrhagic	Traumatic injury Coagulation deficiencies

TABLE 8-4. Summary of Laboratory Findings in Joint Disorders[14,25,35]

Group Classification	Laboratory Findings
I. Noninflammatory	Clear, yellow fluid Good viscosity WBCs less than 5000 Neutrophils less than 30% Normal glucose
II. Inflammatory	Cloudy, yellow fluid Poor viscosity WBCs 2,000 to 100,000 Neutrophils greater than 50% Decreased glucose Possible auto-antibodies present
III. Septic	Cloudy, yellow-green fluid Poor viscosity WBCs 10,000 to 200,000 Neutrophils greater than 90% Decreased glucose Positive culture
IV. Crystal-Induced	Cloudy or milky fluid Poor viscosity WBCs 500 to 200,000 Neutrophils less than 90% Decreased glucose Elevated uric acid Crystals present
V. Hemorrhagic	Cloudy, red fluid Poor viscosity WBCs less than 5000 Neutrophils less than 50% Normal glucose RBCs present

becomes a deeper yellow in the presence of inflammation and may have a greenish tinge with bacterial infection. As with CSF, the presence of blood from a hemorrhagic arthritis must be distinguished from blood due to a traumatic aspiration. This is accomplished primarily by observing the uneven distribution of blood in the specimens obtained from a traumatic aspiration. Turbidity occurs when the cell count is elevated and is usually proportional to the number of cells present. However, a milky fluid may also indicate the presence of crystals.

Viscosity of the synovial fluid comes from the polymerization of the hyaluronic acid and is essential for the proper lubrication of the joints. Arthritis affects both the production of hyaluronate and its ability to polymerize, thus decreasing the viscosity of the fluid. Several methods are used to measure the viscosity of the fluid, the simplest being to visually observe the ability of the fluid to form a string from the tip of a syringe. A string that measures 4 to 6 cm is considered normal. The laboratory may be requested to measure the degree of hyaluronate polymerization by performing a Ropes, or mucin clot, test. When added to a solution of 2 to 5 percent acetic acid, normal synovial fluid will form a solid clot surrounded by clear fluid. As the ability of the hyaluronate to polymerize decreases, the clot becomes less firm and the surrounding fluid increases in turbidity. The Ropes test is reported in terms of good (solid clot), fair (soft clot), poor (friable clot), and very poor (no clot).[42]

Both red and white blood cell counts should be performed on all specimens unless the presence of red blood cells is known to be due to a traumatic tap. Manual counts on thoroughly mixed specimens are done using the Neubauer counting chamber in the same manner as CSF and sperm counts. Clear fluids can usually be counted undiluted, but dilutions are necessary when fluids are turbid or bloody. Dilutions are made in standard Thoma pipettes; however, traditional WBC diluting fluid cannot be used because it contains acetic acid, which will cause the formation of mucin clots. Normal saline can be used as a diluent. If it is necessary to lyse the red blood cells, hypotonic saline or saline that contains saponin are suitable diluents. Methylene blue added to the normal saline will stain the white cell nuclei, permitting separation of the red and white cells during counts performed on mixed specimens. The use of phase rather than light microscopy will also aid in distinguishing between the two cell types.[34] Electronic cell counters are not routinely used for synovial fluid cell counts because the viscous fluid may clog the tubing and the presence of tissue cells can falsely elevate counts. The normal synovial fluid red blood cell count is 0 to 2000 cells per microliter. White blood cell counts below 200 cells per microliter are considered normal and may reach 100,000 cells per microliter or higher in severe inflammations.[29]

Mononuclear cells, including lymphocytes, monocytes, macrophages, and synovial tissue cells, are the primary cells seen in normal synovial fluid. Neutrophils should account for less than 25 percent of the differential count. Increased neutrophils indicate a septic condition; whereas an elevated cell count with a predominance of lymphocytes suggests a nonseptic inflammation. In both normal and abnormal specimens, cells may appear more vacuolated than they do on a blood smear.[24] Besides increased numbers of these usually normal cells, other cell abnormalities include the presence of: LE cells; Reiter cells (vacuolated macrophages with ingested neutrophils); and RA cells, or ragocytes, (neutrophils with small, dark, cytoplasmic granules that consist of precipitated rheumatoid factor).[3,32] Differential counts should be performed on thinly smeared Wright-stained slides; however, an estimate of the percentage of neutrophils present can be obtained from the counting chamber when the diluting fluid contains methylene blue.[24] Table 8-5 summarizes the most frequently encountered cells and inclusions seen in synovial fluid.

Microscopic examination of synovial fluid for the presence of crystals is used in the diagnosis of crystal-induced arthritis. The primary crystals seen in synovial fluid are monosodium urate (uric acid), which is found in cases of gout, and calcium pyrophosphate, which is associated with cases of pseudogout. Cholesterol crystals, crystals of apatite (the major mineral found in cartilage), and corticosteroid crystals resulting from

TABLE 8-5. Cells and Inclusions Seen in Synovial Fluid

Cell/Inclusion	Description	Significance
Neutrophil	Polymorphonuclear leukocyte	Bacterial sepsis Crystal-induced inflammation
Lymphocyte	Mononuclear leukocyte	Non-septic inflammation
Macrophage (Monocyte)	Large mononuclear leukocyte, may be vacuolated	Normal Viral infections
Synovial Lining Cell	Similar to macrophage, but may be multinucleated, resembling a mesothelial cell	Normal
LE Cell	Neutrophil containing characteristic ingested "round body"	Lupus erythematosus
Reiter Cell	Vacuolated macrophage with ingested neutrophils	Reiter's syndrome Nonspecific inflammation
RA Cell (Ragocyte)	Neutrophil with dark cytoplasmic granules containing immune complexes	Rheumatoid arthritis Immunologic inflammations
Cartilage Cells	Large, multinucleated cells	Osteoarthritis
Rice Bodies	Macroscopically resemble polished rice Microscopically show collagen and fibrin	Tuberculosis, septic and rheumatoid arthritis
Fat Droplets	Refractile intracellular and extracellular globules Stain with Sudan dyes	Traumatic injury
Hemosiderin	Inclusions within synovial cells	Pigmented villonodular synovitis

drug injections may also be seen. The microscopic characteristics of these crystals are listed in Table 8-6.

It is recommended that crystal examination be performed soon after the fluid is collected, because changes in temperature and pH in the fluid can affect crystal solubility, producing erroneous results. Refrigeration of specimens decreases the solubility of uric acid, resulting in an increase in monosodium urate crystals. Likewise, a rise in pH due to the loss of carbon dioxide upon exposure to room air encourages the formation of calcium phosphate crystals.[9]

Fluid should be examined unstained, preferably under both direct and compensated polarized light for better visualization and identification of the needle-shaped monosodium urate and calcium pyrophosphate crystals. Monosodium urate crystals are seen routinely as needle-shaped crystals often found within the cytoplasm of neutrophils. Calcium pyrophosphate crystals may appear rhombic-shaped but can also be found as intracellular needles. By examining the refractive properties of the crystals under polarized light, it is possible to differentiate between the two needle-shaped crystals. The basic principle of polarized light is illustrated in Figure 8-4. As can be seen from the

TABLE 8-6. Synovial Fluid Crystals*

Crystal	Shape		Compensated Polarized Light	Location
Monosodium Urate	Needles		Negative birefringence	Intracellular and extracellular
Calcium Pyrophosphate	Rods Needles Rhombics		Positive birefringence	Intracellular and extracellular
Cholesterol	Notched rhombic plates		Negative birefringence	Extracellular
Apatite	Small needles		May need electron microscope	Intracellular and extracellular
Corticosteroid	Flat, variable shaped plates		Positive and negative birefringence	Primarily intracellular

*Adapted from Samuelson and Ward.[39]

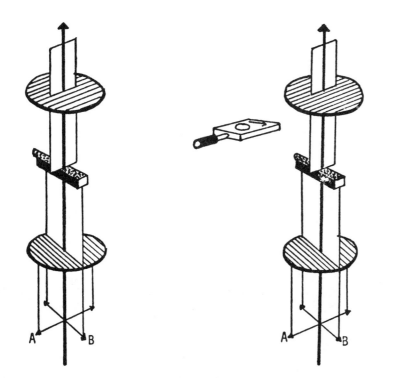

FIGURE 8-4. (*Left*) Direct polarized light. (*Right*) Compensated polarized light. (Adapted from Phelps, Steele, and McCarty.[33])

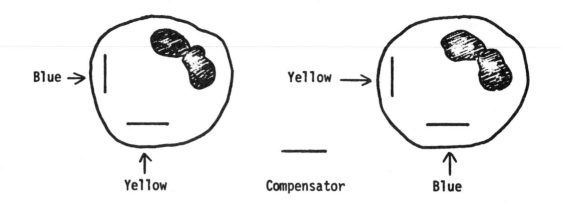

Blue → | Yellow →

Yellow ↑   Compensator   Blue ↑

Monosodium Urate   Calcium Pyrophosphate

FIGURE 8-5. Crystals under compensated polarized light.

diagram, the crystal must be able to bend the light waves (B) that pass through the analyzer. When this happens, the crystal will appear white against a black background. Both monosodium urate and calcium pyrophosphate crystals will polarize direct light; however, monosodium urate will appear brighter against the black background due to its strong birefringence (ability to break the light beam into two rays). Once the presence of crystals has been determined using direct polarized light, positive identification can be made by examining the slide under compensated polarized light. A first-order red compensator is placed in the microscope between the crystal and the analyzer (see Fig. 8-4). The red compensator separates the light beam into slow and fast moving components and retards red light so that the background becomes red instead of black.

Monosodium urate and calcium pyrophosphate crystals exhibit different birefringent properties when light has been separated into slow and fast vibrations, and identification can be made by observing the colors that the crystals produce. When monosodium urate is aligned with the slow vibration, it appears yellow, a sign of negative birefringence; whereas calcium pyrophosphate is blue and positively birefringent. Likewise, when the crystals are aligned opposite the slow vibration, monosodium urate will appear blue and calcium pyrophosphate will appear yellow (Fig. 8-5). Care must be taken to align the crystals in accordance with the direction of slow vibration shown on the compensator. Patterns that vary from those shown in Figure 8-5 may indicate the presence of one of the less common crystals, and additional testing and the patient's history must be considered.

SYNOVIAL FLUID IN THE CHEMISTRY LABORATORY

Since synovial fluid is chemically an ultrafiltrate of plasma, chemistry test values are approximately the same as serum values. Therefore, few chemistry tests are considered clinically important. The most frequently requested test is the glucose determination because markedly decreased values are indicative of inflammatory (Group II) or septic (Group III) disorders. Because normal synovial fluid glucose values are based on the blood glucose level, simultaneous blood and synovial fluid samples should be obtained, preferably after the patient has fasted for 8 hours to allow equilibration between the two fluids. Under these conditions, normal synovial fluid glucose should not be more than 10 mg per dl lower than the blood value.[14]

Recently, measurement of synovial fluid lactate levels has been shown to provide rapid differentiation between inflammatory and septic arthritis and does not require equilibration and comparison with blood lactate levels. Synovial fluid lactate levels below

7.5 mmole per liter provide a 98 percent exclusion for septic arthritis; whereas levels above 7.5 mmole per liter are found consistently with septic arthritis, but may also be seen in rheumatoid arthritis.[7]

Other chemistry tests that may be requested are the total protein and uric acid determinations. Since the large protein molecules are not filtered through the synovial membranes, normal synovial fluid contains less than 3 g per dl of protein (approximately one third of the serum value). Increased levels are found in inflammatory and hemorrhagic disorders; however, measurement of synovial fluid protein does not contribute greatly to the classification of these disorders.[25] When requested, the analysis is performed using the same methods as are used for serum protein determinations. The elevation of serum uric acid in cases of gout is well known; therefore, demonstration of an elevated synovial fluid uric acid may be used to confirm the diagnosis when the presence of crystals cannot be demonstrated in the fluid.

In some laboratories, the performance of the Ropes viscosity test, discussed in the hematology section, is the responsibility of the chemistry department, as is the observation of spontaneous clotting when unheparinized specimens are received.

SYNOVIAL FLUID IN THE MICROBIOLOGY LABORATORY

Although the primary role of the microbiology laboratory is to identify the organisms causing septic inflammations, Gram stains and cultures should be performed on all synovial fluid specimens because infection may occur as a secondary complication of any inflammation.[24] Bacterial infections are most frequently seen; however, fungal, tubercular, and viral infections can also occur. When they are suspected, special culturing procedures should be utilized. Routine bacterial cultures should always include an enrichment media, such as chocolate agar, because in addition to *Staphylococcus* and *Streptococcus,* the most common genera that infect synovial fluid are the fastidious *Hemophilus* and *Neisseria.*

SYNOVIAL FLUID IN THE SEROLOGY LABORATORY

Due to the association of the immune system in the inflammation process, the serology laboratory plays an important role in the diagnosis of joint disorders. However, the majority of the tests are performed on serum, with actual analysis of the synovial fluid serving as a confirmatory measure in cases that are difficult to diagnose. The autoimmune diseases rheumatoid arthritis and lupus erythematosus cause very serious inflammation of the joints and are diagnosed in the serology laboratory by demonstrating the presence of their particular auto-antibodies in the patient's serum. These same antibodies can also be demonstrated in the synovial fluid, if necessary.

Determination of synovial fluid complement levels can be an aid in the differential diagnosis of arthritis as to immunologic and nonimmunologic origin. Measurement of the complement components C1q, C4, C2, and C3 is performed primarily by single radial immunodiffusion.[30] Under normal and nonimmunologic conditions, synovial fluid complement levels parallel the fluid protein levels. Therefore, to ensure that abnormal complement levels are not due to changes in synovial membrane filtration, complement values must be expressed as their ratio to synovial fluid protein.[4]

SEROUS FLUIDS

The closed cavities of the body, namely, the pleural, pericardial, and peritoneal cavities, are each lined by two membranes referred to as the serous membranes. One membrane lines the cavity wall (parietal membrane), and the other covers the organs within the cavity (visceral membrane). The fluid between the membranes, which provides lubrication as the surfaces move against each other, is called serous fluid. Normally, only a small amount of serous fluid is present because production and reabsorption take place at a constant rate.

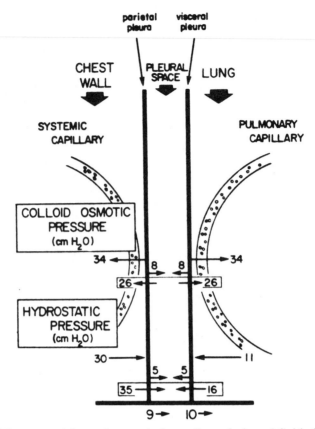

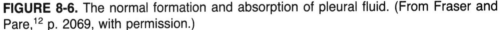

FIGURE 8-6. The normal formation and absorption of pleural fluid. (From Fraser and Pare,[12] p. 2069, with permission.)

FORMATION

Serous fluids are formed as ultrafiltrates of plasma, with no additional material contributed by the membrane cells. The small amount of filtered protein is removed by the lymphatic system. Production and reabsorption are subject to hydrostatic and colloidal (oncotic) pressures from the capillaries servicing the cavities. Under normal conditions, colloidal pressure from serum proteins is the same in the capillaries on both sides of the membrane. Therefore, the greater hydrostatic pressure in the systemic capillaries on the parietal side favors fluid production through the parietal membrane and reabsorption through the visceral membrane. Figure 8-6 demonstrates the normal formation and absorption of pleural fluid.

Fluids for laboratory examination are collected by needle aspiration from the respective cavities. These aspiration procedures are referred to as thoracentesis (pleural), pericardiocentesis (pericardial), and paracentesis (peritoneal). Abundant fluid is usually collected; therefore, suitable specimens are available for each section of the laboratory. An anticoagulated specimen is needed for cell counts, a sterile tube for culture, and a nonanticoagulated specimen for observation of spontaneous clotting. Large volumes of fluid should be concentrated prior to microbiologic and cytologic examinations.

TRANSUDATES AND EXUDATES

Many pathologic conditions can cause a buildup (effusion) of serous fluid. However, a general classification of the cause of the effusion can be accomplished by separating the fluid into the category of transudate or exudate. Effusions that form because of a systemic disorder that disrupts the balance in the regulation of fluid filtration and reabsorption, such as the changes in hydrostatic pressure created by congestive heart

TABLE 8-7. Laboratory Differentiation of Transudates and Exudates

	Transudate	Exudate
Appearance	Clear	Cloudy
Specific Gravity	<1.015	>1.015
Total Protein	<3.0 g/dl	>3.0 g/dl
Fluid:Serum Protein Ratio	<0.5	>0.5
Lactic Dehydrogenase	<200 IU	>200 IU
Fluid:Serum LD Ratio	<0.6	>0.6
Cell Count	<1000/μl	>1000/μl
Spontaneous Clotting	No	Possible

failure, are called transudates. Exudates are produced by conditions that directly involve the membranes of the particular cavity, including infections and malignancies. Transudates can also be thought of as resulting from a mechanical process, and exudates from an inflammatory process. Classification of a serous fluid as to transudate or exudate can provide a valuable initial step in the diagnosis and treatment of the patient.

A variety of laboratory tests have been used to differentiate between transudates and exudates, including appearance, specific gravity, total protein, lactic dehydrogenase, cell counts, and spontaneous clotting. Differential values for these parameters are shown in Table 8-7.

As can be seen using these criteria, one would expect a transudate to be a clear fluid with a specific gravity less than 1.015, protein less than 3.0 g per dl, and a lactic dehydrogenase below 200 IU.

Traditionally, specific gravity and protein were considered to be the most valuable criteria for classification. But in recent years, the lactic dehydrogenase has replaced the specific gravity.[27] Fluid to blood ratios for protein and lactic dehydrogenase have provided greater reliability in the differentiation.[20] As shown in Table 8-8, a combination of the fluid to blood protein ratio, lactic dehydrogenase, and fluid to blood lactic dehydrogenase ratio can provide 100 percent fluid to blood reliability.

GENERAL LABORATORY PROCEDURES

Routine fluid examination, including classification as a transudate or exudate, appearance, cell count and differential, and chemistry and microbiology procedures, is performed in the same manner on all serous fluids. However, the significance of the test results and the need for specialized tests vary among fluids; therefore, the interpretation of routine and special procedures will be discussed individually for each of the three serous fluids.

Cell counts are usually performed manually using the Neubauer counting chamber and the methods discussed in Chapter 7. When performing white cell counts on grossly bloody specimens with high protein levels, the red cells should be lysed using hypotonic saline or saline with saponin. This will prevent any unusual clumping or clotting of the fluid. Some laboratories use electronic cell counters, and good correlation is usually obtained when the cell count is over 1000 cells per μl.[24] Corrections must be made for the inclusion of tissue cells in the count, and care must be taken to prevent the blocking of tubing with fluid debris. Differential counts are performed on Wright-stained smears. The cytologic examination of fluids for the presence of malignant cells is often the most valuable test performed, and it should be performed in the cytology laboratory or by the pathologist.

TABLE 8-8. Classification of Exudates and Transudates*

Criteria	Exudate		Transudate	
	Correct	Misdiagnosed	Correct	Misdiagnosed
Specific gravity 1.016	55 (87.3%)	8 (2.7%)	29 (78.3%)	8 (21.7%)
Pleural fluid protein 3G%	57 (90.4%)	6 (9.6%)	32 (86.4%)	5 (13.6%)
Pleural fluid protein and blood protein ratio 0.5	59 (93.6%)	4 (6.4%)	36 (97.3%)	1 (2.7%)
Pleural fluid LDH and blood LDH ratio 0.6	56 (88.8%)	7 (11.2%)	35 (94.6%)	2 (5.4%)
Pleural fluid LDH 200 I. U.	45 (73.0%)	18 (27.0%)	36 (97.3%)	1 (2.7%)
Pleural fluid glucose 90 mgm%	42 (66.6%)	21 (33.4%)	35 (94.6%)	2 (5.4%)
Pleural fluid WBC-1000	48 (77.9%)	15 (22.1%)	30 (81.0%)	7 (19.0%)
Protein ratio|LDH	61 (96.8%)	2 (3.2%)	37 (100.0%)	0
Protein ratio|LDH ratio	59 (93.6%)	4 (6.4%)	36 (97.3%)	1 (2.7%)
Protein ratio|LDH|LDH ratio	63 (100.0%)	0	37 (100.0%)	0

*From Jain, Gupta, and Kahn,[20] p. 824, with permission.

PLEURAL FLUID

Formation

Abnormal accumulation of pleural fluid (or any serous fluid) will occur when conditions that affect capillary hydrostatic pressure, colloidal pressure, or permeability and lymphatic drainage are present. Examples in each of these cases include congestive heart failure, hypoalbuminemia, pneumonia, and carcinoma.[37] Congestive heart failure and hypoalbuminemia are systemic disorders that result in production of transudate fluid; whereas pneumonia and carcinoma cause localized damage with exudative effusions. Therefore, differentiation of the fluid into the category of transudate or exudate can be significant.

Appearance

Considerable diagnostic information concerning the etiology of a pleural effusion can be learned from the appearance of the specimen. Normal and transudate pleural fluids are clear and pale yellow. Turbidity is usually related to the presence of white blood cells and indicates bacterial infection, tuberculosis, or an immunologic disorder, such as rheumatoid arthritis. The presence of blood in the pleural fluid can signify a hemothorax (traumatic injury), membrane damage such as occurs in malignancy, or may be due to a traumatic aspiration. As is seen with other fluids, blood from a traumatic tap

TABLE 8-9. Pleural Fluid Characteristics in Common Diseases*

Etiology	Appearance	Total WBC (per μl)	Predominant WBC	RBC (per μl)	Protein	Glucose	LDH	Amylase	pH
Transudates									
Congestive heart failure	Clear, straw-colored	<1000	M	0–1000	PF/S <0.5	PF = S	PF/S <0.6 <200 IU/liter	≤S	>7.40
Cirrhosis	Clear, straw-colored	<500	M	<1000	PF/S <0.5	PF = S	PF/S <0.6 <200 IU/liter	≤S	>7.40
Exudates									
Parapneumonic (uncomplicated)	Turbid	5,000–25,000	P	<5000	PF/S >0.5	PF = S	PF/S >0.6	≤S	>7.30
Empyema	Turbid to purulent	25,000–100,000	P	<5000	PF/S >0.5	0–60 mg/dl PF/S <0.5	PF/S >0.6 some >1000 IU/liter	≤S	<7.30
Pulmonary infarction	Straw-colored to bloody	5,000–15,000	P	1,000–100,000	PF/S >0.5	PF = S	PF/S >0.6	≤S	>7.30
Tuberculosis	Straw-colored to serosanguinous	5,000–10,000	M	<10,000	PF/S >0.5	PF = S or <60 mg/dl	PF/S >0.6	≤S	< or >7.30
Rheumatoid disease	Turbid, green to yellow	1,000–20,000	M or P	<1000	PF/S >0.5	<30 mg/dl	Often >1000 IU/liter	≤S	<7.30
Carcinoma	Turbid to bloody	<10,000	M	1,000 to several 100,000	PF/S >0.5	PF = S or <60 mg/dl	PF/S >0.6	≤S	< or >7.30
Pancreatitis	Turbid	5,000–20,000	P	1,000–10,000	PFS >0.5	PF = S	PF/S >0.6	PF/S >2	>7.30

*From Sahn,[36] p. 106–107, with permission.
WBC = White blood cells, RBC = red blood cells, LDH = lactic dehydrogenase, M = mononuclear, PF = pleural fluid, S = serum, IU = international units, P = polymorphonuclear.

appears streaked and uneven. To differentiate between a hemothorax and hemorrhagic exudate, it is necessary to run a hematocrit on the fluid. If the blood is from a hemothorax, the fluid hematocrit will be similar to the whole blood hematocrit because the effusion is actually occurring from the inpouring of blood from the injury. A chronic membrane disease effusion will contain both blood and increased pleural fluid, resulting in a much lower hematocrit.[24] The appearance of a milky pleural fluid may be due to the presence of chylous material from thoracic duct leakage or to pseudochylous material produced in inflammatory conditions. To distinguish between the two substances, the fluid is mixed with ether. True chylous material will be extracted into the ether, leaving a clear layer of fluid.[25]

White blood cell and differential counts are routinely performed on pleural fluids and are useful in the diagnosis of tuberculosis and bacterial infections. Counts above 1000 cells per μl are considered elevated.[24] Tubercular effusions show moderately elevated counts with a predominance of lymphocytes. In bacterial infections, the count is usually higher, and neutrophils are the predominant cell. Increased lymphocytes are also frequently seen in malignant effusions.[28] Although cytologic examination is usually requested separately, the differential smear should be examined for the presence of both normal and abnormal cells. Besides the normal and abnormal cells seen on blood differentials, pleural fluid specimens may also contain macrophages, histiocytes, mesothelial cells, and malignant tissue cells. Mesothelial cells from the pleural membranes can appear in a variety of forms. They are increased in nonseptic inflammations, but are seldom seen in tuberculosis and bacterial infections. Care must be taken not to confuse mesothelial cells with malignant cells, and any questionable cells should be referred to the pathologist.

Since pleural fluid is strictly a plasma ultrafiltrate, normal chemistry values are the same as the plasma levels. Besides the chemical tests used to differentiate transudates and exudates, the most common chemical tests performed on pleural fluid are glucose, pH, and amylase. Decreased glucose levels are seen in tubercular and rheumatoid inflammations. The demonstration of a low fluid pH is of some value in the diagnosis of pneumonia. The finding of a pH as low as 6.0 indicates an esophageal rupture.[11] As with serum, elevated amylase levels are associated with pancreatic disorders; however, amylase is often first elevated in the pleural fluid. Therefore, amylase determinations are recommended procedures on all pleural fluids of questionable etiology. Table 8-9 summarizes the laboratory results for some of the more frequently encountered pleural effusions.

Serologic testing of pleural fluid is used to differentiate effusions of immunologic and malignant origin from those of noninflammatory and nonmalignant origin. The testing includes quantitation of immunoglobulins, complement components, and carcinoembryonic antigen (CEA). Increased levels of immunoglobulins and CEA or decreased complement is indicative of inflammatory and neoplastic reactions. Increased CEA levels provide the best diagnostic information because they are closely associated with malignancy.[1]

PERICARDIAL FLUID

Normally, only a small amount (10 to 50 ml) of clear, pale yellow fluid is found between the pericardial membranes.[25] Pericardial effusions are primarily the result of changes in the permeability of the membranes due to infection (pericarditis), malignancy, or metabolic damage. The presence of an effusion is suspected when cardiac compression is noted during the physician's examination.

Aspirated fluid will appear clear in metabolic disorders. However, turbid fluids, which are produced by infection and malignancy, are more commonly encountered. Milky fluid is seen when damage to the lymphatic system has occurred. Blood-streaked fluid is frequently present when membrane damage is caused by tuberculosis and tumors. Grossly bloody effusions are seen in cardiac puncture and misuse of anticoagulant drugs.

White blood cell counts over 1000 cells per μl are indicative of infection. As with pleural fluid, an increased percentage of neutrophils suggests a bacterial endocarditis.[25] Cytologic examination of pericardial fluid for the presence of malignant cells is an important part of the fluid analysis. Decreased glucose levels are found with bacterial infections and malignancies. Gram stains and cultures are not routinely performed unless bacterial endocarditis is suspected.

PERITONEAL FLUID

Accumulation of fluid in the peritoneal cavity is called ascites, and the fluid is commonly referred to as ascitic fluid rather than peritoneal fluid. Both transudates and exudates occur, and normal saline is sometimes introduced into the peritoneal cavity to act as a lavage for the detection of abdominal injuries that have not yet resulted in the accumulation of fluid. Analysis of lavage fluid is a particularly sensitive test for the detection of intra-abdominal bleeding.[21]

Like pleural and pericardial fluids, normal peritoneal fluid is clear and pale yellow. Exudates are turbid and may appear green when bile is present. The presence of bile can be confirmed using standard chemical screening tests for bilirubin, including urine dipsticks and ferric chloride spot tests. Chylous or pseudochylous material may also be present.

Normal red blood cell counts are usually below 100,000 cells per μl. Elevated counts may indicate hemorrhagic trauma. Should the fluid appear visually bloody, it may not be necessary to perform an actual count. Normal white blood cell counts are below 300 cells per μl, and the count increases with bacterial peritonitis and cirrhosis. To distinguish between these two conditions, an absolute granulocyte count should be performed. An absolute granulocyte count greater than 250 cells per cubic milliliter is indicative of infection.[22] Cytologic examination for malignant cells is, of course, a very important procedure; and as discussed under pleural fluid, measurement of fluid CEA levels can provide valuable diagnostic information in malignancy.[1]

Chemical examination of ascitic fluid consists primarily of glucose, amylase, and alkaline phosphatase determinations. Glucose is decreased below serum levels in tubercular peritonitis and abdominal malignancy. Amylase is routinely determined on ascitic fluid to ascertain cases of pancreatitis, and it may also be elevated in gastrointestinal perforations. An elevated alkaline phosphatase is also highly diagnostic of intestinal perforation. Measurements of blood urea nitrogen and creatinine in the fluid are requested when there is concern about a ruptured bladder or accidental puncture of the bladder during the paracentesis procedure.[15]

Gram stains and bacterial cultures for both aerobes and anaerobes are performed when bacterial peritonitis is suspected, and acid-fast stains and cultures for tuberculosis may also be requested.

AMNIOTIC FLUID

Although much of the current interest in amniotic fluid is in the field of cytogenetics, several very significant tests are performed in the routine clinical laboratory and are discussed in this section.

Amniotic fluid is found in the membranous sac that surrounds the fetus and provides a cushion to protect the fetus (Fig. 8-7). The fluid is formed from the metabolism of fetal cells, transfer of water across the placental membrane, and in later stages of development, by fetal urine. However, by the time production of fetal urine occurs, the fetus begins swallowing the amniotic fluid in an amount approximately equal to the urine output. Therefore, the buildup of amniotic fluid to a total volume of 500 to 2500 ml at term is produced primarily by increased cell metabolism and placental water exchanges. Inability of the fetus to swallow is a critical sign and is indicated by an abnormal increase in amniotic fluid.[16]

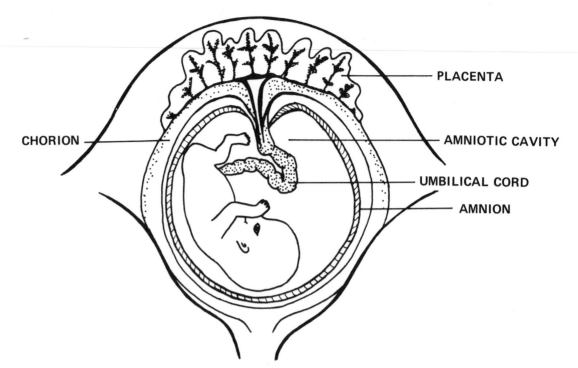

FIGURE 8-7. Fetus in amniotic sac.

Fluid for analysis is obtained by needle aspiration into the amniotic sac, a procedure called amniocentesis. The procedure is relatively safe and can be performed on an outpatient basis. Specimens should be protected from light and promptly delivered to the laboratory. Special precautions must be taken with specimens for cytogenetic analysis because the cells in the fluid must be kept alive for culturing by the laboratory. A 20-ml fluid sample may contain as few as 10 cells! If cell culturing cannot be done immediately, the specimen should be incubated at 37°C for no longer than 2 days. Specimens that must be transported for analysis should be sent by express, courier-delivered mail to ensure prompt delivery.

Clinical analysis of amniotic fluid assesses both fetal well-being and maturation. Since amniotic fluid is a product of fetal metabolism, the constituents that are present in the fluid provide information about the metabolic processes taking place and the progress of fetal maturation. When conditions that adversely affect the fetus arise, the danger to the fetus must be measured against the ability of the fetus to survive an early delivery.

The oldest and still most routinely performed laboratory test on amniotic fluid evaluates the severity of the fetal anemia produced by hemolytic disease of the newborn. In lay terms, these infants are referred to as "Rh babies." The incidence of this disease has been decreasing rapidly since the development of methods to prevent anti-Rh antibody production in postpartum mothers. However, the problem does and will continue to exist, so laboratory personnel must be prepared to analyze these specimens. The destruction of fetal red blood cells by antibodies that are present in the maternal circulation results in the appearance of the red blood cell degradation product, bilirubin, in the amniotic fluid. By measuring the amount of bilirubin present in the fluid, it is possible to determine the degree of hemolysis taking place and to assess the danger this anemia presents to the fetus.

The measurement of amniotic fluid bilirubin is performed by spectrophotometric analysis. As illustrated in Figure 8-8, the optical density of the fluid is measured in intervals between 365 mμ and 550 mμ, and the readings are plotted on semilogarithmic graph paper. In normal fluid, the optical density will be highest at 365 mμ and will decrease linearly (Plot A) to 550 mμ. However, when bilirubin is present, a rise in optical density

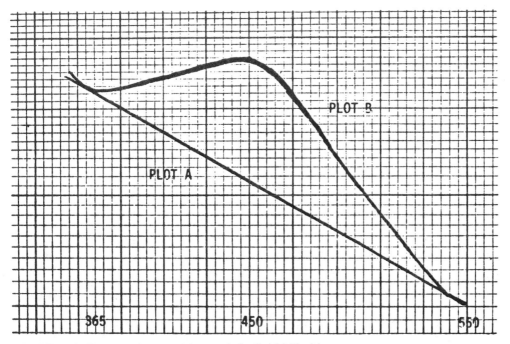

FIGURE 8-8. Spectrophotometric amniotic fluid bilirubin scans.

will be seen at 450 mμ because this is the wave length of maximum bilirubin absorption (Plot B). The amount of bilirubin present can be determined from the height of the peak, thereby providing a measure of the degree of red cell destruction. Extreme care must be taken to protect the specimen from light, since bilirubin is a very light-sensitive chemical and markedly decreased values will be obtained with as little as 30 minutes of exposure to light.[16]

Fetal distress, whether caused by hemolytic disease of the newborn or other conditions, forces the obstetrician to consider a preterm delivery. At this point, it becomes necessary to assess fetal maturity. Respiratory distress is the most frequent complication of early delivery. Therefore, laboratory tests are performed to determine the maturity of the fetal lung, as well as the overall fetal maturity.

The laboratory procedure routinely used to measure fetal lung maturity is the lecithin-sphingomyelin ratio (L/S ratio). Lecithin is the primary component of the phospholipids that make up the majority of the alveolar lining and account for alveolar stability. Lecithin is produced at a relatively low and constant rate until the 35th week of gestation, at which time a noticeable increase in its production occurs, resulting in the stabilization of the fetal lung alveoli. Sphingomyelin is a lipid that is produced at a constant rate throughout fetal gestation; therefore, it can serve as a control on which to base the rise in lecithin. Both lecithin and sphingomyelin appear in the amniotic fluid in amounts proportional to their concentrations in the fetus.[17] Prior to 35 weeks of gestation, the L/S ratio is usually less than 1.6, and it will rise to 2.0 or higher when lecithin production increases. Therefore, when the L/S ratio reaches 2.0, a preterm delivery is usually considered to be a relatively safe procedure.[46]

A more exact evaluation of fetal lung maturity can be made by performing a lung profile, in which the concentrations of not only lecithin and sphingomyelin but also the other lung surface lipids, phosphatidylglycerol, phosphatidylinositol, and desaturated lecithin, are measured.[26] Absence of phosphatidylglycerol in the presence of a normal L/S ratio is seen in children of diabetic mothers; and even though phosphatidylglycerol represents only 10 percent of the lung surface lipids, respiratory distress will occur if it is not present.[18] No correlation between the presence or absence of phosphatidylinositol and the occurrence of respiratory distress has been demonstrated.[41] However, because

TABLE 8-10. Tests for Fetal Well-being and Maturity

Test	Normal Values at Term[16]	Significance
Bilirubin Scan	0.025 mg/dl	Hemolytic disease of the newborn
L/S Ratio	2.0	Fetal lung maturity
Phosphatidylglycerol	Present	Fetal lung maturity
Creatinine	1.8–4.0 mg/dl	Fetal age
Alpha Fetal Protein	4.0 mg/dl	Neural tube disorders

the appearance of phosphatidylinositol in amniotic fluid parallels that of lecithin, measurement of phosphatidylinositol and phosphatidylglycerol may be used in place of the L/S ratio when fluid has been contaminated with serum, which contains lecithin but not phosphatidylinositol or phosphatidylglycerol.[19] Measurement of lung surface lipids is performed using thin-layer chromatography.[31]

Until the development of thin-layer chromatography techniques to measure the individual lung surface lipid concentrations, a mechanical screening test, called the "foam" or "shake" test, was used to determine their presence. Because it can be performed at the bedside or in the laboratory, the test is still in use. Amniotic fluid is mixed with 95 percent ethanol, shaken for 15 seconds, and then allowed to sit undisturbed for 15 minutes. At the end of this time, the surface of the fluid is observed for the presence of a continuous line of bubbles around the outside edge. The presence of bubbles correlates well with fetal lung maturity, although the analysis is more subjective than the L/S ratio.[10] A more recently developed procedure for measuring the total amniotic fluid lung surface lipid concentration is based on the ability of lecithin, phosphatidylglycerol, and phosphatidylinositol to decrease the polarized fluorescence produced by 1,6-diphenyl-1,3,5-hexatriene. However, specialized instrumentation is required to perform this test.[6]

Fetal age can be determined by measuring the amount of creatinine in the amniotic fluid. At about 36 weeks of gestation, urine from the fetal kidney begins appearing in the amniotic fluid; therefore, a creatinine concentration above 2.0 mg per dl indicates a fetal age of approximately 36 weeks.[45] As more is learned about the role of the fetal metabolites that are present in the amniotic fluid in the assessment of fetal well-being and maturity, additional chemical tests will become part of the amniotic fluid analysis. Already, the measurement of alpha fetal protein levels and acetylcholinesterase activity is being used to provide early detection of neural tube disorders, such as spina bifida and anencephaly.[2] Table 8-10 summarizes the routine chemical tests performed on amniotic fluid.

Cytogenetic analysis of amniotic fluid, although not performed in the routine clinical laboratory, has become an important predictor of hereditary birth defects. Chromosomal analysis for the presence of Down's syndrome in the fetuses of women over 35 has become a common procedure, and amniocentesis is routinely performed on women who have a family history of genetic defects. As would be expected, the performance of cytogenetic analyses on the amniotic fluid is a controversial subject.

SWEAT

Although the analysis of sweat is not a frequently requested clinical laboratory procedure, measurement of the sweat electrolytes, sodium and chloride, is performed to confirm the diagnosis of cystic fibrosis. Cystic fibrosis is a metabolic disease that affects the mucus-secreting glands of the body. It is inherited as an autosomal recessive and is seen in approximately 1 out of every 1500 to 2000 Caucasian births.[43] Because cystic fibrosis involves multiple organs, many clinical symptoms can lead the physician to suspect its presence. The most common indicators include family history of cystic fibrosis, newborns who fail to thrive or who have intestinal obstructions, and the appearance of pancreatic insufficiency or respiratory distress in infants. The demonstration of elevated sweat sodium and chloride values in patients who exhibit any or all of these symptoms serves to confirm the diagnosis of cystic fibrosis.

Proper collection and handling of sweat specimens can present a problem for the laboratory when one considers that the patient, often an infant, must be induced to sweat and that the sweat produced cannot be aspirated into a collection tube. Earlier methods to stimulate the production of sweat, including the use of humid, high-temperature rooms and encasing the patient's body in plastic, have currently been replaced by Gibson and Cooke's[40] pilocarpine iontophoresis technique. Sweat glands on the forearm are subjected to the sweat-inducing alkaloid pilocarpine in the presence of a mild electrical current. Following stimulation, the area is thoroughly cleansed, and using forceps, preweighed electrolyte-free gauze or filter paper is placed on the stimulated area and tightly sealed to prevent evaporation. Using pilocarpine iontophoresis, a sufficient amount of sweat for analysis can be collected in 25 to 30 minutes. After reweighing the pads to determine the amount of sweat collected, the sweat is eluted using a measured amount of deionized water.

Recently, comparisons between sweat electrolytes and sweat osmolarity have shown good correlation. After pilocarpine iontophoresis stimulation, a vapor pressure osmometer pad is placed directly on the surface and sealed with plastic. Because the sweat osmolarity is measured on an undiluted sample, care must be taken to include the water that condenses on the plastic cover, or values will be falsely elevated.[44]

The actual collection of the sweat can be avoided by applying a chloride electrode to the skin following stimulation and measuring the concentration directly. However, since the amount of sodium present should approximate the chloride concentration, most laboratories prefer to measure both parameters to provide better quality control for the procedure.[43] The method may also produce inaccurate readings in the high ranges when influenced by air bubbles and temperature fluctuations.[44]

Chloride is measured by automatic or manual titration methods and sodium by flame photometry or ion exchange electrodes. Sweat chloride and sodium values over 70 mEq per liter are seen consistently in 98 percent of patients with cystic fibrosis and are almost never found in normal individuals. Concentrations over 40 mEq per liter are considered borderline, and the test should be repeated at a later date if the patient's clinical symptoms so warrant.[40] Early diagnosis of cystic fibrosis is most important for prolonged patient survival.

REFERENCES

1. BERTI, P, ET AL: *Diagnostic value of glycoproteins, immunoglobulin, complement and CEA in pleural and peritoneal effusions.* Quad Sclavo Diagn 17(4):483–494, 1981.
2. BROCK, DJH: *Prenatal diagnosis: Chemical methods.* Br Med Bull 32(1):16–19, 1976.
3. BRODERICK, PA, ET AL: *Exfoliative cytology: Interpretation of synovial fluid in disease.* J Bone Joint Surg 58-A(3):396–399, 1976.
4. BUNCH, TW, ET AL: *Synovial fluid complement determination as a diagnostic aid in inflammatory joint disease.* Mayo Clin Proc 49:715–720, 1974.
5. CANNON, DC: *Examination of the seminal fluid.* In HENRY, JB (ED): *Clinical Diagnosis and Management by Laboratory Methods.* WB Saunders, Philadelphia, 1984.
6. CHESKIN, HS AND BLUMENFELD, TA: *Evaluation of fetal lung maturity by measure-*

ment of 1,6-diphenyl-1,3,5-hexatriene fluorescence polarization in amniotic fluid. Clin Chem 27(11):1934–1937, 1981.

7. CURTIS, G, NEWMAN, R, AND SLACK, M: *Synovial fluid lactate and the diagnosis of septic arthritis.* Journal of Infection 6:239–246, 1983.

8. CZUPPON, AB AND METTLER, I: *Estimation of anti-spermatozoa antibody concentrations by a* [125]*I protein-A binding assay in sera of infertile patients.* J Clin Chem Clin Biochem 21(6):357–362, 1983.

9. DIEPPE, P, ET AL: *Laboratory handling of crystals.* Ann Rheum Dis (Suppl) 42:60–63, 1983.

10. DOVER, JS AND ELLIOT, HC: *Unidimensional chromatographic determination of phosphatidyl glycerol and L/S ratio with predictive values for L/S ratio, phosphatidyl glycerol and foam stability index.* Laboratory Medicine 13(3):159–161, 1982.

11. DYE, RA AND LAFORET, EG: *Esophageal rupture: Diagnosis by pleural fluid pH.* Chest 66(4):454–456, 1974.

12. FRASER, RG AND PARE, JAP: *Diagnosis of Disease of the Chest, Vol. 1.* WB Saunders, Philadelphia, 1977.

13. GLASSER, L: *Seminal fluid and subfertility.* Diagnostic Medicine 4(5):28–45, 1981.

14. GLASSER, L: *Body fluid analysis: Synovial fluid.* Diagnostic Medicine 3(4):35–50, 1980.

15. GLASSER, L: *Body fluid evaluation: Serous fluids.* Diagnostic Medicine 3(5):79–90, 1980.

16. GLASSER, L: *Amniotic fluid and the quality of life.* Diagnostic Medicine 4(6):31–51, 1981.

17. GLUCK, L, ET AL: *Diagnosis of the respiratory distress syndrome by amniocentesis.* Am J Obstet Gynecol 109(3):440–445, 1971.

18. HALLMAN, M, ET AL: *Absence of phosphatidyl glycerol (PG) in respiratory distress syndrome in the newborn.* Pediatr Res 11(6):714–720, 1977.

19. HALLMAN, M, ET AL: *Phosphatidylinositol and phosphatidylglycerol in amniotic fluid: Indices of lung maturity.* Am J Obstet Gynecol 125(5):613–617, 1976.

20. JAIN, AP, GUPTA, OP, AND KHAN, N: *Comparative diagnostic efficiency of criteria used for differentiating transudate and exudate pleural effusions.* J Assoc Physicians India 30(11):823–825, 1982.

21. JERGENS, ME: *Peritoneal lavage.* Am J Surg 133:365–369, 1977.

22. JONES, SR: *The absolute granulocyte count in ascites fluid: An aid to the diagnosis of spontaneous bacterial peritonitis.* West J Med 126(5):344–346, 1977.

23. KEEL, BS: *The semen analysis: An important diagnostic evaluation.* Laboratory Medicine 10(11):686–688, 1979.

24. KJELDSBERG, CR AND KNIGHT, JA: *Body Fluids, Laboratory Examination of Cerebrospinal, Synovial and Serous Fluids: A Textbook Atlas.* American Society of Clinical Pathologists, Chicago, 1982.

25. KJELDSBERG, CR AND KRIEG, A: *Cerebrospinal fluid and other body fluids.* In HENRY, JB (ED): *Clinical Diagnosis and Management by Laboratory Methods.* WB Saunders, Philadelphia, 1984.

26. KULOVICH, MV, HALLMAN, MB, AND GLUCK, L: *The lung profile: Normal pregnancy.* Am J Obstet Gynecol 135:57–60, 1979.

27. LIGHT, R, ET AL: *Pleural effusions: The diagnostic separation of transudates and exudates.* Ann Intern Med 77:507–513, 1971.

28. LIGHT, RW, EROZAN, YS, AND BALL, WC: *Cells in pleural fluid: Their value in differential diagnosis.* Arch Intern Med 132:854–860, 1973.

29. NAIB, ZM: *Cytology of synovial fluids.* Acta Cytol 17(4):299–309, 1973.

30. OCHI, T, YONEMASU, K, AND ONO, K: *Immunochemical quantitation of complement components of C1q and C3 in sera and synovial fluid of patients with bone and joint diseases.* Ann Rheum Dis 39(3):235–240, 1980.

31. PAPPAS, AA, MULLINS, RE, AND GADSDEN, RH: *Improved one-dimensional thin-layer chromatography of phospholipids in amniotic fluid.* Clin Chem 28(1):209–211, 1982.

32. PEKIN, RJ, MALININ, TI, AND ZVAIFLEN, NJ: *Unusual synovial fluid findings in Reiter's syndrome.* Ann Intern Med 66(4):677–684, 1967.

33. PHELPS, P, STEELE, AD, AND MCCARTY, DJ: *Compensated polarized light microscopy: Identification of crystals in synovial fluid from gout and pseudogout.* JAMA 203(7):166–171, 1968.

34. REVILL, PA: *Examination of synovial fluid.* Curr Top Pathol 71:2–24, 1982.

35. RIPPEY, J: *Synovial fluid analysis.* Laboratory Medicine 10(3):140–145, 1979.

36. SAHN, SA: *Pulmonary diseases.* In RELLER, LB, SAHN, SA, AND SCHRIER, RW (EDS): *Clinical Internal Medicine.* Little, Brown & Co, Boston, 1979.

37. SAHN, SA: *The differential diagnosis of pleural effusions.* West J Med 137(2):99–108, 1982.

38. SAMPSON, JH AND ALEXANDER, NJ: *Semen analysis: A laboratory approach.* Laboratory Medicine 13(4):218–223, 1982.

39. SAMUELSON, CO AND WARD, JR: *Examination of the synovial fluid.* J Fam Pract 14(2):343–349, 1982.

40. SHWACHMAN, H AND MAHMOODIAN, A: *The sweat test and cystic fibrosis.* Diagnostic Medicine 5(4):61–77, 1982.

41. SKJAERAASEN, J AND STRAY-PEDERSEN, S: *Amniotic fluid phosphatidylinositol and phosphatidylglycerol: Normal pregnancy.* Acta Obstet Gynecol Scand 58:225–229, 1979.

42. TELOH, HA: *Clinical pathology of synovial fluid.* Ann Clin Lab Sci 5(4):282–287, 1975.

43. TOCCI, PM AND MCKEY, RM: *Laboratory confirmation of the diagnosis of cystic fibrosis.* Clin Chem 22(11):1841–1844, 1976.

44. WEBSTER, HL: *Laboratory diagnosis of cystic fibrosis.* CRC Crit Rev Clin Lab Sci 18(4):313–337, 1983.

45. WEISS, RR, ET AL: *Amniotic fluid uric acid and creatinine as measures of fetal maturity.* Obstet Gynecol 44(2):208–214, 1974.

46. WENT, RE, ROSENBAUM, J, AND STATLAND, BE: *Amniotic fluid and antenatal diagnosis.* In HENRY, JB (ED): *Clinical Diagnosis and Management by Laboratory Methods.* WB Saunders, Philadelphia, 1984.

STUDY QUESTIONS (Choose one best answer)

1. Proper collection of a semen specimen should include all of the following except:

    a. collection in a sterile container
    b. collection after a 3-day period of sexual abstinence
    c. collection at the laboratory followed by 1 hour of refrigeration
    d. collection at home and delivery to the laboratory within 1 hour

2. Semen specimens should be analyzed:

    a. immediately upon receipt
    b. prior to liquefaction
    c. after liquefaction
    d. one hour after collection

3. An abnormal amount of prostatic fluid in a semen specimen will:

    a. lower the pH
    b. raise the pH
    c. increase the viscosity
    d. decrease the viscosity

4. The normal sperm count is:

   a. 140 to 200 million per microliter
   b. 50 to 100 million per milliliter
   c. 40 to 160 million per milliliter
   d. 50 to 100 million per microliter

5. The purpose of diluting semen specimens with sodium bicarbonate and formalin prior to counting is to:

   a. ensure liquefaction of the specimen
   b. allow motility to be determined while performing the count
   c. enhance the cellular morphology
   d. immobilize and preserve the sperm

6. The motility component of a sperm analysis includes all of the following except:

   a. differentiation between progressive and brownian movement
   b. determination of the percentage of motile sperm
   c. determination of the quality of movement
   d. differentiation between motility of normal and abnormal sperm

7. An acceptable percentage of abnormal sperm after examination of 200 cells is:

   a. zero
   b. less than 10%
   c. less than 30%
   d. less than 50%

8. A normal semen analysis followed by continued infertility may be the result of:

   a. decreased concentration of fructose
   b. decreased sperm viability
   c. sperm agglutinins in the male
   d. sperm agglutinins in the female

9. Semen analysis on post-vasectomy patients should be performed:

   a. within 1 week
   b. one month post-vasectomy
   c. until two consecutive monthly specimens show no sperm
   d. until two consecutive monthly specimens show no viable sperm

10. The presence or absence of semen in a specimen can accurately be determined by testing for:

    a. fructose
    b. alkaline phosphatase
    c. acid phosphatase
    d. agglutinating antibodies

11. All of the following statements on synovial fluid are true except:

    a. it surrounds all joints in the body
    b. it is found only in the knee

c. it acts as a lubricant
d. it supplies nourishment to cartilage

12. Which of the following descriptions of synovial fluid does not match:

    a. normal = clear, pale yellow
    b. crystals = milky
    c. traumatic tap = blood streaks
    d. sepsis = uniform blood

13. In the Ropes, or mucin clot, test, normal synovial fluid:

    a. forms a solid clot when added to hydrochloric acid
    b. forms a solid clot when added to glacial acetic acid
    c. forms a friable clot when added to hydrochloric acid
    d. forms a friable clot when added to glacial acetic acid

14. A white blood cell count on synovial fluid obtained during a traumatic tap should be diluted with:

    a. glacial acetic acid and methylene blue
    b. 0.1N hydrochloric acid and methylene blue
    c. normal saline and methylene blue
    d. hypotonic saline and methylene blue

15. Neutrophils that contain precipitated rheumatoid factor in their cytoplasm are called:

    a. LE cells
    b. Reiter cells
    c. ragocytes
    d. macrophages

16. Synovial fluid for crystal examination should be:

    a. stained with Wright's stain and examined with bright-field microscopy
    b. stained with methylene blue and examined under polarized light
    c. examined unstained under direct and compensated polarized light
    d. examined unstained with bright-field microscopy

17. Crystals found in synovial fluid during attacks of gout are:

    a. monosodium urate
    b. calcium pyrophosphate
    c. cholesterol
    d. apatite

18. Examination of synovial fluid under direct polarized light reveals intracellular needle-shaped crystals that appear white against the black background. When a red compensator is added and the crystals are aligned with the slow vibration, they appear yellow against the red background. These crystals are:

    a. monosodium urate showing positive birefringence
    b. monosodium urate showing negative birefringence
    c. calcium pyrophosphate showing positive birefringence
    d. calcium pyrophosphate showing negative birefringence

19. Crystals that appear extracellularly as rhombic-shaped and intracellularly as needle-shaped and are blue when aligned with the slow vibration of compensated polarized light are:

    a. monosodium urate
    b. calcium pyrophosphate
    c. apatite
    d. corticosteroid

20. In gout, both serum and synovial fluid will have increased levels of:

    a. glucose
    b. protein
    c. uric acid
    d. complement

21. A cloudy, yellow-green synovial fluid with 100,000 WBCs, a predominance of neutrophils, and a decreased glucose would be classified as:

    a. noninflammatory
    b. inflammatory
    c. septic
    d. crystal-induced

22. An arthrocentesis performed on a patient with lupus erythematosus produces a cloudy yellow fluid with 2000 WBCs, of which 55% are neutrophils. This fluid would be classified as:

    a. noninflammatory
    b. inflammatory
    c. septic
    d. crystal-induced

23. Fluid collected by thoracentesis is called:

    a. pleural
    b. pericardial
    c. peritoneal
    d. ascitic

24. Serous fluid effusions may result from all of the following except:

    a. congestive heart failure
    b. hypoalbuminemia
    c. increased capillary permeability
    d. dehydration

25. Effusions produced by conditions that directy affect the serous membranes are termed:

    a. transudates
    b. exudates

26. To be classified as an exudate, a fluid should have:

    a. total protein less than 3 g/dl, specific gravity less than 1.015, and LD less than 200 IU
    b. total protein less than 3 g/dl, specific gravity greater than 1.015, and LD greater than 200 IU
    c. total protein greater than 3 g/dl, specific gravity greater than 1.015, and LD greater than 200 IU
    d. total protein greater than 3 g/dl, cell count less than 1000/μl, and fluid to serum LD ratio less than 0.6

27. Differentiation between a hemothorax and a hemorrhagic exudate on a bloody pleural fluid is done by:

    a. observing the fluid for streaks of blood, because this indicates a hemothorax
    b. performing a hematocrit, because a hemothorax will give a value similar to the whole blood
    c. performing an RBC count, because a hemorrhagic effusion will have a count over 100,000/μl
    d. performing both RBC and WBC counts, because a hemothorax will have marked elevations of both cell types

28. A milky pleural fluid becomes clear after extraction with ether. This fluid contained:

    a. chylous material from thoracic duct leakage
    b. pseudochylous material from thoracic duct leakage
    c. chylous material from inflammation
    d. pseudochylous material from inflammation

29. A pleural fluid pH of less than 6.0 is indicative of:

    a. tuberculosis
    b. malignancy
    c. pancreatic disorders
    d. esophageal rupture

30. Peritoneal lavage is performed to:

    a. remove ascitic fluid
    b. check for the presence of bile
    c. detect intra-abdominal bleeding
    d. provide a sufficient volume of fluid for chemical analysis

31. Requests for amylase and alkaline phosphatase determinations on ascitic fluid are received in suspected cases of:

    a. peritonitis
    b. gastrointestinal perforations
    c. ruptured bladder
    d. malignancy

32. Amniotic fluid is formed by all of the following except:

    a. fetal urine
    b. fetal cell metabolism

c. fetal swallowing

d. transfer of water across the placenta

33. An amniocentesis is performed on a woman whose last two pregnancies have resulted in stillbirths due to hemolytic disease of the newborn. A screening test performed at the hospital is positive for bilirubin, and the specimen is sent to a reference lab for a bilirubin scan. Doctors are concerned when the report comes back negative, and they question if:

a. the correct specimen was sent

b. the specimen was refrigerated

c. the specimen was exposed to light

d. the specimen reached the reference lab within 30 minutes

34. Tests to determine the maturity of the fetal lung and overall fetal maturity are:

a. bilirubin, L/S ratio, and creatinine

b. bilirubin, L/S ratio, and phosphatidylglycerol

c. creatinine, L/S ratio, and phosphatidylglycerol

d. L/S ratio and phosphatidylglycerol

35. The foam, or shake, test is a screening test for amniotic fluid:

a. bilirubin

b. L/S ratio

c. alpha fetal protein

d. phosphatidylglycerol

36. Sweat electrolytes run on specimens collected by pilocarpine iontophoresis are:

a. elevated in muscular dystrophy

b. elevated in cystic fibrosis

c. decreased in cystic fibrosis

d. decreased in muscular dystrophy

⑨
GASTRIC ANALYSIS

INSTRUCTIONAL OBJECTIVES

Upon completion of this chapter, readers will be able to:

1. describe the production and composition of the gastric secretion

2. differentiate between total acidity and titratable acidity

3. calculate the milliequivalents per liter of titratable acid when provided with the appropriate titration data

4. calculate the acid output, maximum acid output, and peak acid output when provided with the appropriate titration data

5. state the normal volume, acid output, and significance of the basal gastric analysis

6. discuss the advantages and disadvantages of the pentagastrin, histamine, Histalog, and insulin stimulation tests

7. describe the typical post-stimulation gastric analysis results in hyperacidity and pernicious anemia

8. define anacidity

Due to the development of non-laboratory procedures for the evaluation of gastric function which are considered more precise, less time-consuming, and less uncomfortable for the patient, routine examination of gastric contents by the clinical laboratory has been diminishing. Of major interest in the laboratory analysis of gastric secretion is the measurement of gastric acidity, which has been considered useful in the diagnosis and treatment of peptic ulcers, gastric carcinoma, and pernicious anemia. Additional procedures now in use for the detection of these disorders include direct examination of lesions by endoscopy, improved radiologic techniques, pH sensitive electrodes that will transmit pH readings when passed into the stomach, measurement of serum gastrin levels, cytologic examination of gastric contents for malignant cells, and immunologic testing of serum for the presence of anti–intrinsic factor and anti–parietal cell antibodies seen in pernicious anemia.[1] The sophistication of these procedures has reduced the diagnostic role of actual gastric acidity titration to a secondary one in many instances. However, since the analysis is still requested by some physicians, students should be instructed in the performance and significance of the procedure and its relationship to other examinations currently being utilized.

PHYSIOLOGY

Gastric acidity results from the secretion of hydrochloric acid by the parietal cells in the stomach. These cells are also responsible for the production of intrinsic factor necessary for the intestinal absorption of vitamin B_{12}. Hydrochloric acid converts the enzyme precursor pepsinogen, secreted by the zymogen chief cells, to the enzyme pepsin, which catalyzes the digestion of protein. Stimulation of the parietal cells to produce acid is caused primarily by the hormone gastrin, which is secreted by specialized G cells in the lower portion of the stomach. Neurologic stimulation by the vagus nerve and the presence of food and fluid in the stomach promote the G cells to secrete gastrin. Besides the two major components, hydrochloric acid and pepsin, gastric secretions may also contain saliva, mucus, acid neutralizing chemicals, and material regurgitated from intestinal, biliary, and pancreatic secretions.

SPECIMEN COLLECTION

Gastric contents are collected by nasal or oral intubation of the patient. To ensure complete collection of gastric secretions, the position of the tube is checked by fluoroscopic examination of the stomach. Patients should be instructed not to swallow excessive amounts of saliva during the collection period, because saliva will neutralize the gastric acidity. Collection is usually performed on patients in the fasting state. A more complete recovery of the gastric contents is obtained if aspiration is performed continuously throughout the collection period. However, because acidity testing is routinely performed on 15-minute specimens, the aspiration must be collected in time-labeled containers that represent each 15 minutes of the required collection period, and not as a single specimen.

OLD TITRATION PROCEDURE

Routine tests performed on gastric specimens include volume, pH, and titratable acidity. Different theories have existed concerning the types of acids present and their significance in the disease process. For many years, it was believed that acid with a pH of less than 3.5 represented "free" or hydrochloric acid, and that the remainder of the acid present below pH 8.4 was "combined" or organic acid. The two acids were measured separately by titrating the specimen first with 0.1N NaOH, using the indicator Töpfer's reagent, which changes from red to yellow at pH 3.5. Then the titration was continued using phenolphthalein as an indicator and titrating from colorless to a faint pink color that appears at approximately pH 8.4. The titration using Töpfer's reagent represented the hydrochloric acid present; the titration with phenolphthalein measured the organic acid. The sum of the two titrations determined the total acidity of the specimen. The results were reported in "degrees of acidity," which represented the number of milliliters of 0.1N NaOH that were needed to titrate 100 ml of gastric secretion to the end point of the indicator being used (3.5 with Töpfer's reagent, and 8.4 with phenolphthalein).[3]

CURRENT TITRATION PROCEDURE

Current theories question the existence of two distinct gastric acid phases and recommend the measurement of the overall hydrogen ion concentration. Therefore, both the ionized and un-ionized hydrogen are measured simultaneously by titrating the specimen with 0.1N NaOH to pH 7.0 using the indicator phenol red, which changes from yellow to red in the pH range 6.0 to 7.4. Titration results are reported as milliequivalents or millimoles per liter of titratable acid, rather than in "degrees of acidity." This is a more conventional manner of test reporting, although, as can be seen from the definition of "degrees of acidity," the numerical results will be the same. Milliequivalents per liter of titratable acid are calculated from the amount of 0.1N NaOH needed to reach the phenol red end point using the standard formula $C_1 \times V_1 = C_2 \times V_2$.

Example: Calculate the milliequivalents per liter of titratable acid in a 20-ml specimen when 2.0 ml of 0.1N NaOH are used to reach pH 7.0.

$$0.1N \ NaOH \times 2 \ ml = X \times 20 \ ml$$
$$20X = 0.2$$
$$X = 0.01 \ equivalents/liter$$
$$0.01 \ equivalents/liter \times 1000 = 10 \ mEq/liter$$

Notice that when 0.1N is used in the calculation, the answer is in equivalents per liter and must be changed to milliequivalents per liter by multiplying by 1000. This can be avoided by converting the 0.1N NaOH to 100 mEq or 100 mmole prior to performing the calculation.

Since titratable acidity represents the milliequivalents or millimoles of acid per liter, and the typical gastric secretion specimen is of considerably less volume, it also becomes necessary to calculate the actual acid output in the specimen. This is done by multiplying the specimen volume in liters by the titratable acidity.

Example: The first 15-minute specimen of a 1-hour basal collection has a volume of 25 ml. To titrate 10 ml of this specimen to the end point of phenol red, 5 ml of 0.1N NaOH are used. Calculate the titratable acidity and the acid output of the specimen.

A. $100 \ mEq/liter \ NaOH \times 5 \ ml = X \times 10 \ ml$
   $10X = 500 \ mEq/liter$
   $X = 50 \ mEq/liter \ titratable \ acid$

B. $\dfrac{25 \ ml \ specimen}{1000 \ ml} \times 50 \ mEq/liter = 1.25 \ mEq \ acid/specimen$

BASAL GASTRIC ACIDITY

The above example refers to the basal, or fasting, specimen, which is the initial collection in the gastric analysis. The basal specimen is a 1-hour collection, usually consisting of four 15-minute specimens, although any other time frame may be used, including a single 1-hour collection. The volume, pH, titratable acidity, and acid output of the samples that constitute the basal specimen are determined. Normal values for volume and acidity are based on the total 1-hour specimen. Therefore, individual sample results must be combined to provide the 1-hour total. A wide variety of normal values for the basal gastric secretion can be found throughout the literature; however, in general, the normal basal secretion has a volume of about 30 to 60 ml and contains a low acid output of approximately 1.0 to 4.0 mEq per hour.[1] Besides providing a baseline upon which to compare subsequent test results, the major diagnostic value of the basal gastric analysis lies in the finding of markedly elevated acidity. This is indicative of the Zollinger-Ellison syndrome, a condition of gastric hypersecretion produced by a gastrin-secreting tumor of the pancreas.

POST-STIMULATION GASTRIC ACIDITY

The inability to produce gastric acidity cannot be solely determined from the analysis of the basal gastric secretion; therefore, additional tests must be performed. Several test variations are available, but all utilize the same principle, which is to introduce a gastric stimulant into the patient following the basal collection. Specimens continue to be collected and are tested for increased volume and acid content. Commonly used stimulants include pentagastrin, histamine, and Histalog. The stimulant of choice is currently pentagastrin, a synthetic compound resembling gastrin, because it does not

TABLE 9-1. Sample Gastric Analysis*

Specimen #		Specimen Volume	Volume Titrated	M1 0.1N NaOH Used	Titratable Acidity (mEq/liter)	Acid Output (mEq)	Basal Acid Output (mEq/hr)	Maximum Acid Output (mEq/hr)	Peak Acid Output (mEq/hr)
Basal	#1	10	10	2.2	22	0.22			
	#2	15	10	2.0	20	0.30			
	#3	20	10	1.5	15	0.30			
	#4	5	5	2.5	50	0.25	1.07		
Stimulated	#1	30	10	6.5	65	1.95			
	#2	50	10	12.5	125	6.25			
	#3	50	10	13.0	130	6.50			Times 2
	#4	40	10	11.5	115	4.60		19.3	25.5

*Analysis of four 15-minute basal specimens and four 15-minute specimens collected following administration of pentagastrin.

TABLE 9-2. Representative Normal and Abnormal Gastric Analysis Results[1,4]

	Basal Acid Output (mEq/hr)	Maximum Acid Output (mEq/hr)	BAO/MAO
Normal	2.5	25.0	10%
Pernicious Anemia	0	0	0
Gastric Carcinoma	1.0	4.0	25%
Duodenal Ulcer	5.0	30.0	17%
Zollinger-Ellison Syndrome	18.0	25.0	72%

cause the patient the discomfort that occurs with histamine administration, and it produces a more rapid response than Histalog. When pentagastrin or histamine is utilized as the stimulant, specimens are collected at 15-minute intervals for 1 hour following the injection. When Histalog is administered, the collection must continue for 2 hours because maximum acid output is delayed. A 2-hour collection of both basal and post-stimulation samples is required when performing the insulin hypoglycemia test used to determine if surgical removal of the vagus nerve has been successful. Insulin stimulation of the parietal cells to produce acid is transmitted by the vagus nerve; therefore, a successful vagotomy will prevent the production of hyperacidity in response to insulin.[2]

All post-stimulation specimens are analyzed in the same manner as the basal specimens, by measuring volume, pH, and titratable acidity, and calculating acid output. The hourly acid output is calculated and is referred to as the maximum acid output in post-stimulation tests. Some laboratories consider calculation of the peak hourly acid output to be a more reproducible parameter. Peak acid output is determined by taking the total of the two highest 15-minute acid outputs and multiplying this figure by two to arrive at the hourly acid output.[1] When pentagastrin or histamine is administered, the peak acidity is usually seen within 15 to 45 minutes post-injection; whereas with Histalog, the peak appears between 45 and 75 minutes. An example of a complete gastric secretion analysis, including titratable acidity, acid output, maximum acid output, and peak acid output, is shown in Table 9-1. Normal values are again highly variable; however, normal individuals will usually not produce a maximum acid output over 40 mEq.[1] Persons who are unable to produce gastric acidity, as is seen in pernicious anemia and some cases of gastric carcinoma, show no response to the stimulation, and the pH of the specimens does not fall below 6.0. Normal individuals will exhibit a fall in pH to below 3.5. Hourly basal and maximum acid outputs that are representative of conditions that produce abnormal gastric acidity are provided in Table 9-2.

TERMINOLOGY

Just as the theories concerning the significance and performance of the gastric analysis have changed, so has the terminology used to describe the variations in gastric acidity. The terms anacidity, achlorhydria, and hypochlorhydria have all been used to describe the inability to produce gastric acid. However, since their definitions were originally based on the distinction made between "free" and "combined" acid and the titration to pH 3.5, the use of three different terms has been abandoned. Only the term anacidity has been retained to designate the inability to produce gastric acid, and it is defined as failure to produce a pH of less than 6.0 following gastric stimulation.[2]

SUMMARY

In summary, it appears that although the gastric analysis still holds a small role in the clinical laboratory, its value will probably continue to decline as more sophisticated procedures are developed and perfected.

REFERENCES

1. BARON, JH: *Clinical Tests of Gastric Secretion: History, Methodology and Interpretation.* Macmillan, London, 1978.
2. CANNON, DC: *Examination of gastric and duodenal contents.* In HENRY, JB (ED): *Clinical Diagnosis and Management by Laboratory Methods.* WB Saunders, Philadelphia, 1984.
3. FREEMAN, JA AND BEELER, MF: *Laboratory Medicine: Urinalysis and Medical Microscopy.* Lea & Febiger, Philadelphia, 1983.
4. MARKS, IN, ET AL: *The augmented histamine test: A review of 615 cases of gastroduodenal disease.* S Afr J Surg 1:53–59, 1963.

STUDY QUESTIONS (Choose one best answer)

1. Gastric acidity is produced as the result of:

   a. stimulation of the zymogen chief cells by gastrin to produce hydrochloric acid
   b. stimulation of the parietal cells by gastrin to produce hydrochloric acid
   c. stimulation of the parietal cells by signals from the vagus nerve
   d. stimulation of specialized G cells by pepsinogen to produce hydrochloric acid

2. The major constituents of gastric secretions are:

   a. hydrochloric acid and mucus
   b. hydrochloric acid and bile
   c. hydrochloric acid and saliva
   d. hydrochloric acid and pepsin

3. Falsely decreased values for gastric acidity will occur if:

   a. the patient is intubated while fasting
   b. the patient swallows large amounts of saliva
   c. the aspiration is performed continuously over the collection period
   d. the patient receives Histalog during the collection period

4. The recommended method of measuring gastric acidity is:

   a. titrate with 0.1N NaOH to pH 3.5 with Töpfer's reagent, and report in degrees of acidity
   b. titrate with 0.1N NaOH to pH 3.5 with Töpfer's reagent, and report in milliequivalents per liter
   c. titrate with 0.1N NaOH to pH 7.0 with phenol red, and report in degrees of acidity
   d. titrate with 0.1N NaOH to pH 7.0 with phenol red, and report in milliequivalents per liter

5. At pH 7.0, phenol red changes from:

   a. yellow to red
   b. red to yellow
   c. colorless to red
   d. red to colorless

6. Calculate the milliequivalents per liter of titratable acidity in a 15-ml specimen if 3.0 ml of 0.1N NaOH are used to titrate 10 ml to pH 7.0.

7. The above specimen represents the first 15-minute collection in a 1-hour basal specimen. Calculate the actual acid output of the specimen.

8. All 15-minute specimens of a 1-hour basal specimen produce results identical to those of the specimen in Question 6. You would interpret this specimen to be:

   a. indicative of Zollinger-Ellison syndrome
   b. indicative of pernicious anemia
   c. indicative of an improperly collected specimen
   d. indicative of normal gastric acidity

9. The preferred stimulant of gastric acidity for routine analysis is:

   a. histamine
   b. Histalog
   c. pentagastrin
   d. insulin

10. Post-stimulation specimens from persons with pernicious anemia will show:

    a. no increased acidity and a pH above 6.0
    b. no increased acidity but a pH below 6.0
    c. increased acidity and a pH below 6.0
    d. increased acidity and a pH below 3.5

11. Post-stimulation specimens for maximum acid output are:

    a. collected, analyzed, and reported the same as basal specimens
    b. collected as a total 1-hour specimen, which is analyzed and reported as milli-equivalents of acid output
    c. collected in the same manner as basal specimens but analyzed only for pH
    d. collected as a 1-hour specimen and analyzed for degrees of acidity

12. The inability to produce gastric acidity and a pH of less than 6.0 is termed:

    a. achlorhydria
    b. hypochlorhydria
    c. anacidity
    d. hypoacidity

10
FECAL ANALYSIS

INSTRUCTIONAL OBJECTIVES
Upon completion of this chapter, readers will be able to:

1. describe the normal composition of feces

2. name a pathogenic and nonpathogenic cause, when presented with an abnormal description of fecal color

3. state the significance of increased neutrophils in a stool specimen

4. name the fecal fats stained by Sudan III and give the conditions under which they will stain

5. describe and interpret the microscopic results that will be seen when a specimen from a patient with steatorrhea is stained with Sudan III

6. state the principle of the chemical screening tests for "occult" blood

7. discuss the advantages and disadvantages of ortho-tolidine and guaiac as substrates in the "occult" blood screening test

8. briefly describe a chemical test performed on feces for each of the following: steatorrhea, fetal hemoglobin, pancreatic insufficiency, and carbohydrate intolerance

In the minds of most laboratory personnel, analysis of fecal specimens fits into the category of a "necessary evil." Indeed, as an end-product of body metabolism, feces do provide necessary diagnostic information. Routine fecal examination includes macroscopic, microscopic, and chemical analyses for the early detection of gastrointestinal bleeding, liver and biliary duct disorders, and malabsorption syndromes. Of equal diagnostic value is the detection and identification of pathogenic bacteria and parasites; however, these procedures are best covered in a microbiology textbook and will not be discussed here.

SPECIMEN COLLECTION
Collection of fecal specimens is seldom an easy task for the patient. Containers should be provided and patients instructed to collect the specimen in a clean container, such as a bedpan, and then to transfer the specimen to the laboratory container. They should be cautioned to avoid mixing the specimen with urine or contaminating it with water from the toilet because it may contain chemical disinfectants. Specimens received in the laboratory vary from material collected on a physician's glove to 3-day specimens collected in paint cans. Small random specimens are adequate for performing quali-

tative tests for blood and microscopic examination for white blood cells and undigested materials, such as protein fibers and fecal fat. However, for quantitative analysis, timed specimens are needed in order to measure daily output. Due to the variability in bowel habits, the most representative timed sample is a 3-day collection.

PHYSIOLOGY

The normal fecal specimen contains bacteria, cellulose and other undigested foodstuffs, gastrointestinal secretions, bile pigments, cells from the intestinal walls, electrolytes, and water. Many species of bacteria make up the normal flora of the intestines and contribute to the digestive process. Bacterial metabolism produces the strong odor associated with feces. Disruption of the normal intestinal flora will lead to diarrhea, as will the introduction of pathogenic organisms. Digestive enzymes are secreted into the intestine primarily by the pancreas and function in the breakdown and absorption of proteins, carbohydrates, and fats. Major enzymes include trypsin, chymotrypsin, aminopeptidase, and lipase for the degradation of fats. Lack of one of these enzymes will cause an inability to digest and absorb a particular foodstuff, resulting in the appearance of excess undigested material in the feces and the clinical symptoms of a malabsorption syndrome. Bile salts contribute to the digestion of fats; and bile pigment, in the form of urobilin, is believed to provide the normal brown color of the feces. Consequently, obstruction of the flow of bile into the intestine will lead to the production of light colored, fatty stools. Water and electrolytes are readily reabsorbed in the intestinal tract, and under normal conditions, the electrolyte concentration of the feces approximates that of the plasma. Should the intestinal contents become highly concentrated, excess water will remain in the intestine and diarrhea will result. Constipation, on the other hand, provides time for additional water to be reabsorbed from the fecal material, producing small, hard stools.

The section of the laboratory to which routine fecal analysis is assigned varies among hospitals. Most commonly, the screening of random samples is included with the cultures and parasitology in microbiology or is performed in urinalysis. Quantitative analyses are performed in the chemistry section.

FECES IN THE URINALYSIS LABORATORY

Routine fecal tests performed in the urinalysis laboratory include: macroscopic observation of the color and consistency; microscopic examination for white blood cells, protein fibers, and fecal fat; and qualitative chemical tests for blood.

COLOR AND APPEARANCE

The first indication of gastrointestinal disturbances can often be provided by changes in the normal brown color of the feces. Of course, the appearance of abnormal fecal color may also be caused by the ingestion of highly pigmented foods and medications, so a differentiation must be made between this and a possible pathologic cause. Most frequently referred to is the black, tarry stool associated with upper gastrointestinal bleeding. Blood originating from the esophagus, stomach, or duodenum takes approximately 3 days to appear in the stool; during this time, degradation of hemoglobin produces the characteristic black color. Likewise, blood from the lower gastrointestinal tract requires less time to appear and will retain its original red color. Both black and red stools should be chemically tested for the presence of blood because ingestion of iron will often produce a black stool and many foods and medications contain red pigment. The appearance of pale stools can also cause concern; however, the recent administration of barium should first be considered, since this is a frequent nonpathogenic reason for grayish white stools. If barium has not been ingested, obstruction of the flow of bile pigment to the intestine and the lack of enzymes necessary for the digestion and absorption of fat must be investigated. In cases of fat malabsorption, termed steatorrhea, the stools are often bulky and frothy and may appear pale or dark

TABLE 10-1. Macroscopic Stool Characteristics[2,7]

Appearance	Possible Cause
Black	Upper gastrointestinal bleeding Iron therapy Charcoal Bismuth
Red	Lower gastrointestinal bleeding BSP dye Pyridium compounds Beets and food coloring
Pale Yellow, White, Gray	Bile duct obstruction
Yellow	Rhubarb
Green	Biliverdin Green vegetables Antibiotics
Bulky/Frothy	Steatorrhea
Ribbon-like	Intestinal constriction
Mucus	Constipation Malignancy Colitis

yellow. Stools from suspected cases of steatorrhea should be tested for the presence of excess fat. Besides variations in color, additional abnormalities that may be observed during the macroscopic examination include the watery consistency present in diarrhea, and the small, hard stools seen with constipation. Slender, ribbon-like stools suggest an obstruction of the normal passage of material through the intestine. Also, the presence of mucus may indicate inflammation of the intestinal walls, and blood-streaked mucus shows excessive irritation to the walls. A summary of the major macroscopic abnormalities is given in Table 10-1.

WHITE BLOOD CELLS

Microscopic examination of the feces for the presence of white blood cells is performed as a preliminary procedure in determining the cause of diarrhea. Neutrophils are seen in the feces in conditions that affect the intestinal wall, such as ulcerative colitis and infection with invasive bacterial pathogens. Organisms that cause diarrhea by toxin production, rather than intestinal wall invasion, do not cause the appearance of neutrophils in the feces. Therefore, the presence or absence of fecal neutrophils can provide the physician with diagnostic information prior to the isolation of a bacterial pathogen. As few as three neutrophils per high-power field can be indicative of an invasive condition.[2] Specimens may be examined as wet preparations stained with methylene blue, or they may be stained with Gram or Wright's stains.

QUALITATIVE FECAL FATS

Specimens from suspected cases of steatorrhea can be microscopically screened for the presence of excess fecal fat. Although this is a qualitative procedure that should be followed by a quantitative chemical measurement of fecal fat concentration, there is good correlation between the two procedures when the microscopic examination is carefully performed.[8] Lipids are found in the feces primarily in the form of neutral fats (triglycerides), fatty acid salts (soaps), and fatty acids. Their presence can be microscopically observed by staining with the dyes Sudan III, Sudan IV, or oil red O, of which Sudan III is the most routinely used. Neutral fats are readily stained by Sudan III and appear as large orange-red droplets often located near the edge of the coverslip.[9] Observation of more than 60 droplets per high-power field can be considered indicative of steatorrhea.[5] Soaps and fatty acids do not stain directly with Sudan III. Soaps must be converted to fatty acids by acetic acid, and fatty acids need to be melted to absorb the dye. Therefore, a second slide must be examined after the specimen has been mixed with acetic acid and heated. Examination of this slide will reveal stained droplets that represent not only the free fatty acids but also the fatty acids produced by hydrolysis of the soaps and the neutral fats. Normal specimens may contain as many as 100 small droplets, less than 4 microns in size, per high-power field.[4] Larger droplets, often more than 75 microns in size, are commonly seen in steatorrhea. Therefore, not only the number but also the size of the droplets must be considered when evaluating the slide for fatty acid content.[6] The presence of many large droplets may indicate the combination of several fatty acids, which would falsely decrease the droplet count. Comparison of the results obtained from the initial examination representing neutral fat content and the post-hydrolysis slide containing fatty acids can aid in determining if steatorrhea is due to a lack of pancreatic enzymes or a malabsorption disorder. Since pancreatic enzymes break down neutral fats to fatty acids for reabsorption, an increase in neutral fat content indicates a deficiency in pancreatic enzymes. In contrast, steatorrhea caused by a malabsorption disorder would have a normal neutral fat content and increased fatty acids.[1]

OCCULT BLOOD

By far the most frequently performed fecal analysis is the chemical screening test for the detection of "occult," or hidden, blood. As discussed earlier, bleeding in the upper gastrointestinal tract may produce a black, tarry stool, and bleeding in the lower gastrointestinal tract may result in an overtly bloody stool. However, since any bleeding in excess of 2 milliliters per 150 grams of stool is considered pathologically significant, and no visible signs of bleeding may be present with this amount of blood, chemical detection of the "occult" blood is necessary.[3] Originally used primarily to test suspected cases of gastrointestinal disease, the "occult" blood test has currently become widely used as a mass screening procedure for the early detection of colorectal cancer. The "occult" blood test detects 75 percent of colorectal cancers while they are still in the localized stage. This can result in a cure rate of 71 percent, as opposed to 43 percent for nonlocalized cases.[10]

Several different chemicals have been used to detect "occult" blood. All react in the same chemical manner but vary in their sensitivity. Listed in order of decreasing sensitivity, these compounds include benzidine, ortho-tolidine, and gum guaiac. Contrary to most chemical testing, the least sensitive reagent, guaiac, is preferred for routine testing. This choice can be better understood when one considers the chemical reaction taking place. This reaction utilizes the pseudoperoxidase activity of hemoglobin reacting with hydrogen peroxide to oxidize a colorless compound to a colored compound:

$$\text{Hemoglobin} \xrightarrow[\text{peroxidase}]{\text{pseudo-}} H_2O_2 \xrightarrow{O} \begin{array}{c} \text{benzidine} \\ \text{ortho-tolidine} \\ \text{guaiac} \end{array} \longrightarrow \text{blue color}$$

Pseudoperoxidase activity, the key to this reaction, is also present in animal hemoglobin, certain vegetables, and some intestinal bacteria. Therefore, random samples collected from people under no dietary restrictions would produce false-positive reactions if tested with too sensitive a reagent. Benzidine, the most sensitive compound, is no longer available for clinical use because it possesses carcinogenic properties. Both ortho-tolidine and guaiac are available in commercial kits for laboratory use. Hematest (Ames Company, Elkhart, Indiana) supplies ortho-tolidine combined with tartaric acid, calcium acetate, and strontium peroxide in tablet form. When the tablet is placed on a fecal specimen and water is added, the tartaric acid and calcium acetate react with the strontium peroxide, releasing the peroxide to be acted upon by the hemoglobin pseudoperoxidases. If these peroxidases are present in the specimen, a blue color will be produced by the oxidized ortho-tolidine.[5] Because the sensitivity of ortho-tolidine may produce false-positive reactions, this test is most useful for monitoring patients with controlled dietary intake.

The products used in routine mass screening for "occult" blood include Hemoccult (Smith Kline Diagnostics, Sunnyvale, California) and Fecatest (FinnPipette Ky, Helsinki, Finland). Both kits contain guaiac-impregnated filter paper to which the fecal specimen and hydrogen peroxide are added. In the presence of hemoglobin peroxidase activity, a blue color will appear on the impregnated filter paper. Packaging of the guaiac-impregnated filter paper in individually sealed containers has facilitated the mass screening program for colorectal cancer by allowing persons at home to place a portion of the specimen on the paper and mail it to the laboratory for testing. When possible, the fecal specimen placed on the filter paper should represent several portions of the stool, including the center, since intermittent bleeding may produce positive and negative areas in the same stool.[2] Persons collecting specimens at home must be cautioned to avoid contamination of the specimen with toilet bowl cleaners, which may interfere with the peroxidase reaction. Due to the decreased sensitivity of the guaiac reagent, it is recommended that at least three and, ideally, six different specimens be tested before a negative result is confirmed. False-negative results have also been reported from persons taking large doses of vitamin C, and false-positive reactions may occur in conjunction with iron therapy.[3] Additional methods for the detection of "occult" blood are currently under development and include an immunologic test that is specific for human hemoglobin and a chemical test that converts the heme portion of hemoglobin to porphyrin for analysis by fluorescence.[2]

FECES IN THE CHEMISTRY LABORATORY
QUANTITATIVE FECAL FATS

Quantitative chemical analysis of feces in the clinical laboratory is confined primarily to the measurement of fecal fat content for the confirmation of steatorrhea. As discussed earlier, quantitative fecal analysis requires the collection of at least a 3-day specimen. The patient must also maintain a regulated intake of fat prior to and during the collection period. Paint cans make excellent collection containers because the specimen must be homogenized prior to analysis, and this can be accomplished by placing the container on a conventional paint-can shaker. The method routinely used for fecal fat measurement is the Van de Kamer titration.[9] Fecal lipids are converted to fatty acids and titrated to a neutral end point with sodium hydroxide. The fat content is reported as grams of fat or fatty acids per 24 hours. Normal values are based on fat intake and range from 4 to 6 percent of the ingested fat.

APT TEST

Should it be necessary to distinguish between the presence of fetal or maternal blood in an infant's stool or vomitus, the Apt test may be requested. The material to be tested is emulsified in water to release hemoglobin, and after centrifugation, 1 percent NaOH is added to the pink hemoglobin-containing supernatant. In the presence of alkali-resistant fetal hemoglobin, the solution will remain pink; whereas denaturation of the maternal hemoglobin will produce a yellow-brown supernatant.

TRYPSIN

Absence of the protein-digesting enzyme, trypsin, can be screened for by placing a small amount of stool emulsified in water on a piece of X-ray paper. In the presence of trypsin, the gelatin on the X-ray paper will be digested, leaving a clear area on the paper. Inability to digest the gelatin indicates a deficiency in trypsin production and is associated with pancreatic insufficiency. The gelatin test may be requested, in conjunction with more specific tests discussed in Chapter 8, on infants suspected of having cystic fibrosis.

CARBOHYDRATES

Carbohydrate malabsorption or intolerance is primarily analyzed by serum tests; however, an increased concentration of carbohydrate can be detected by performing a copper reduction test on the fecal specimen. Carbohydrate testing is most valuable in assessing cases of infant diarrhea and may be accompanied by a pH determination, because utilization of the increased carbohydrate by intestinal bacteria will produce a lowered pH. The test is performed using a Clinitest tablet (Ames Company, Elkhart, Indiana) and one part stool emulsified in two parts water. As discussed in Chapter 4, this is a general test for the presence of reducing substances, and a positive result would be followed by more specific serum carbohydrate tolerance tests, the most common of these being the D-xylose and lactose tolerance tests.

SUMMARY

A summary of fecal screening tests is presented in Table 10-2.

TABLE 10-2. Summary of Fecal Screening Tests

Test	Methodology/Principle	Interpretation
Examination for Neutrophils	Microscopic count of neutrophils in smear stained with methylene blue, Gram, or Wright's stain	3/hpf indicates condition affecting intestinal wall
Qualitative Fecal Fats	Microscopic examination of direct smear stained with Sudan III	60 large orange-red droplets indicate lack of pancreatic digestive enzymes
	Microscopic examination of smear heated with glacial acetic acid and Sudan III	100 small orange-red droplets or large droplets indicate malabsorption
Occult Blood	Pseudoperoxidase activity of hemoglobin liberates oxygen to oxidize gum guaiac	Blue color indicates gastrointestinal bleeding
Apt Test	Addition of NaOH to hemoglobin-containing emulsion determines presence of maternal or fetal blood	Pink color indicates presence of fetal hemoglobin
Trypsin	Emulsified stool placed on X-ray paper to determine ability to digest gelatin	Inability to digest gelatin indicates lack of trypsin
Clinitest	Addition of emulsified stool to Clinitest to detect presence of reducing substances	Presence of reducing substances suggests carbohydrate malabsorption

REFERENCES

1. ANDERSON, DH: *Celiac syndrome, determination of fat in feces; Reliability of two chemical methods and microscopic estimate; Excretion of feces and of fecal fat in normal children.* Am J Dis Child 69(3):141–151, 1945.
2. BRADLEY, GM: *Fecal analysis: Much more than an unpleasant necessity.* Diagnostic Medicine 3(2):64–75, 1980.
3. CARROLL, S: *Fecal occult blood: Efficacy of testing measures.* Nurse Pract 5(5):15–21, 1980.
4. DRUMMEY, GD, BENSON, JA, AND JONES, CM: *Microscopic examination of the stool for steatorrhea.* N Engl J Med 264:85–87, 1961.
5. FREEMAN, JA AND BEELER, MF: *Laboratory Medicine: Urinalysis and Medical Microscopy.* Lea & Febiger, Philadelphia, 1983.
6. GHOSH, SK, ET AL: *Stool Microscopy in Screening for Steatorrhea.* J Clin Pathol 30:749–753, 1977.
7. KAO, YS AND SCHEER, WD: *Malabsorption, diarrhea, and examination of feces.* In HENRY, JB (ED): *Clinical Diagnosis and Management by Laboratory Methods.* WB Saunders, Philadelphia, 1979.
8. SEMKO, V: *Fecal fat microscopy.* Am J Gastroenterol 75(3):204–208, 1981.
9. VAN DE KAMER, JH, ET AL: *A rapid method for determination of fat in feces.* J Biol Chem 177:347–355, 1949.
10. WINAWER, SJ: *Screening for colorectal cancer: An overview.* Cancer 45(5):1093–1098, 1980.

STUDY QUESTIONS (Choose one best answer)

1. The normal brown color of the feces is produced by:

   a. undigested foodstuffs
   b. urobilin
   c. pancreatic enzymes
   d. cellulose

2. Diarrhea can result from all of the following except:

   a. disruption of the normal intestinal bacterial flora
   b. addition of pathogenic organisms to the normal intestinal flora
   c. increased reabsorption of intestinal water and electrolytes
   d. increased concentration of fecal electrolytes

3. Stools from persons with steatorrhea will contain excess amounts of:

   a. barium sulfate
   b. mucus
   c. blood
   d. fat

4. Which of the following pairings of stool appearance and cause does not match?

   a. black tarry = blood
   b. yellow-green = barium sulfate
   c. pale, frothy = steatorrhea
   d. yellow-white = bile duct obstruction

5. Microscopic examination of stools provides preliminary information as to the cause of diarrhea because:

   a. neutrophils will be present in conditions caused by toxin-producing bacteria
   b. neutrophils will be present in conditions that affect the intestinal wall

c. red and white blood cells will be present if the cause is bacterial

d. lymphocytes will be present if the condition is of nonbacterial etiology

6. Large orange-red droplets seen on direct microscopic examination of stools mixed with Sudan III represent:

   a. fatty acids
   b. soaps
   c. neutral fats
   d. cholesterol

7. Microscopic examination of stools mixed with Sudan III and glacial acetic acid and then heated will show small orange-red droplets that represent:

   a. soaps
   b. fatty acids and soaps
   c. fatty acids and neutral fats
   d. fatty acids, soaps, and neutral fats

8. Examination of direct and post-hydrolysis slides for fat droplets reveals a normal neutral fat content and an increased amount of fatty acids. This is indicative of:

   a. steatorrhea due to increased triglyceride consumption
   b. steatorrhea due to lack of pancreatic enzymes
   c. steatorrhea due to inability to convert fatty acids to soaps
   d. steatorrhea due to a malabsorption disorder

9. The term "occult blood" describes blood that:

   a. is produced in the lower gastrointestinal tract
   b. is produced in the upper gastrointestinal tract
   c. is not visibly apparent in the stool specimen
   d. produces a black, tarry stool

10. Tests for the detection of occult blood rely on the:

    a. reaction of hemoglobin with hydrogen peroxide
    b. pseudoperoxidase activity of hemoglobin
    c. reaction of hemoglobin with ortho-tolidine
    d. pseudoperoxidase activity of hydrogen peroxide

11. Gum guaiac is preferred over ortho-tolidine for occult blood in mass screening tests because:

    a. there is less interference from dietary hemoglobin
    b. ortho-tolidine is less sensitive
    c. gum guaiac reacts equally with formed and watery stools
    d. filter paper is more easily impregnated with gum guaiac

12. In the Van de Kamer method for quantitative fecal fat determinations:

    a. fecal lipids are homogenized and titrated to a neutral end point with sodium hydroxide
    b. fecal lipids are measured gravimetrically after ashing
    c. fecal lipids are converted to fatty acids prior to titrating with sodium hydroxide
    d. fecal lipids are measured by spectrophotometer after addition of Sudan III

APPENDIX
ANSWER KEY

CHAPTER 1

1. c	7. b	13. Glycolysis had occurred; dilute random specimen
2. a	8. d	
3. b	9. b	14. 2-hour postprandial with fasting specimen
4. d	10. c	
5. d	11. d	
6. b	12. b	

CHAPTER 2

1. d	9. d	17. d	25. b
2. d	10. c	18. c	26. c
3. c	11. d	19. b	27. b
4. d	12. a	20. c	28. a
5. b	13. c	21. d	29. d
6. a	14. d	22. b	30. 675 ml/min
7. b	15. 100 ml/min	23. b	31. c
8. d	16. 100 ml/min	24. c	32. e, c, f, a, b

CHAPTER 3

1. c	5. d	9. a	13. b
2. a	6. b	10. d	14. c
3. b	7. a	11. 1.009	15. d
4. c	8. c	12. c	16. a

CHAPTER 4

1. b	10. a	19. d	28. b
2. c	11. c	20. c	29. c
3. c	12. d	21. a	30. b
4. d	13. c	22. b	31. b
5. b	14. a	23. c	32. d
6. a	15. c	24. b	33. c
7. d	16. b	25. d	34. c, e, f, c, c,
8. c	17. b	26. c	d, g, b, f, b
9. d	18. c	27. d	

35. a. yes
    b. no
    c. yes
    d. no

36. a. The patient's clinical symptoms suggest a urinary tract infection. Large doses of ascorbic acid may be interfering with the nitrite and leukocyte tests.
    b. Red blood cell protein would contribute to the urinary protein, as would leukocytes.
    c. Amber urine suggesting a concentrated specimen is also produced by large doses of vitamin A (carotene).
    d. Bacterial breakdown of urine urea to ammonia and vegetarian diets raise urinary pH.

CHAPTER 5

1. c	6. d	11. b	16. d
2. b	7. a	12. b	17. d
3. d	8. b	13. d	18. a
4. a	9. c	14. b	19. d
5. c	10. c	15. b	20. a

21. a. triple phosphate
    b. ammonium biurate
    c. calcium oxalate
    d. calcium carbonate

22. d
    a
    e
    b

23. a. Positive blood and cloudy specimen.
    b. Positive nitrite suggests urinary infection.
    c. Protein and acidic pH provide conditions for cast formation.
    d. Positive nitrite caused by bacterial reduction of urinary nitrate.

24. a. Positive blood; however, RBCs may have lysed in dilute alkaline urine.
    b. Positive nitrite and clinical symptoms suggest urinary infection.
    c. Alkaline pH and small amount of protein do not favor cast formation.
    d. Positive nitrite caused by bacterial reduction of urinary nitrate.

25. Concentrated urine containing casts and RBCs is frequently seen after strenuous exercise. After a period of rest, the results should return to normal.

26. a. Did you recheck the pH and verify crystal identification?
    b. Did you call the result to the physician?
    c. Did the patient have a recent IVP?
    d. Did you confirm reactivity of dipstick, and did you consider yeast or oil droplets?

CHAPTER 6

1. c	7. d	13. c	19. a
2. c	8. a	14. d	20. b
3. d	9. d	15. b	21. d
4. a	10. a	16. b, a, a, b, b	22. b
5. b	11. d	17. c	23. c
6. c	12. d	18. c	

CASE STUDIES

1. A diet high in fresh Hawaiian pineapple would produce a false-positive 5-HIAA. This result would return to normal after dietary restriction.

2. The blue color in the catheter bag could be caused by the oxidation of urinary indican to indigo blue. Bobby's symptoms are consistent with Hartnup disease, which can be controlled by dietary regulation.

3. The ferric chloride tube test and the DNPH test are consistent with phenylketonuria and maple syrup urine disease. False-negative PKU results on first specimens are most frequently seen in female infants; therefore, this test should be repeated and urinary amino acid chromatography should be performed.

CHAPTER 7

1. b	9. c	17. a	25. b
2. c	10. d	18. d	26. d
3. c	11. b	19. b	27. d
4. a, a, b, b	12. a	20. c	28. b
5. c	13. c	21. a	29. b
6. 167/μl	14. b	22. c	30. a
7. a	15. a	23. d	
8. 3000/μl	16. d	24. d	

CASE STUDIES

1. Results suggest a bacterial meningitis. Other tests could include a CSF lactate and a Limulus Lysate test for the presence of gram-negative organisms. There is at least a 10 percent possibility of a false-negative Gram stain and culture. Blood cultures could be helpful.

2. Clinical symptoms and initial test results suggest multiple sclerosis, which can be confirmed with protein electrophoresis and an IgG index.

3. Viral = lactate, LD isoenzymes
   Tubercular = acid-fast stain, lactate, glucose
   Fungal = Gram stain, India ink, lactate, glucose

CHAPTER 8

1. c	10. c	19. b	28. a
2. c	11. b	20. c	29. d
3. a	12. d	21. c	30. c
4. c	13. b	22. b	31. b
5. d	14. d	23. a	32. c
6. d	15. c	24. d	33. c
7. c	16. c	25. b	34. c
8. d	17. a	26. c	35. b
9. c	18. b	27. b	36. b

CHAPTER 9

1. b	4. d	7. 0.3 acid mEq	10. a
2. d	5. a	8. d	11. a
3. b	6. 20 mEq/liter	9. c	12. c

CHAPTER 10

1. b	4. b	7. d	10. b
2. c	5. b	8. d	11. a
3. d	6. c	9. c	12. c

COLOR PLATES

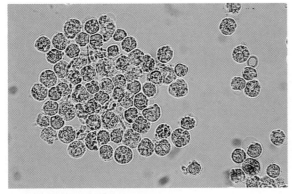

1. White Blood Cells, (400X)

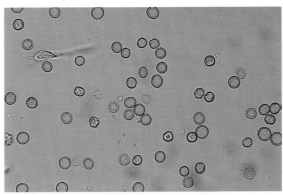

2. Red Blood Cells, (400X)

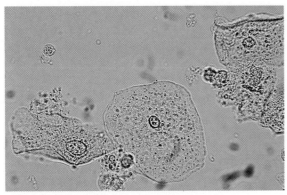

3. Squamous Epithelial Cells, (400X)

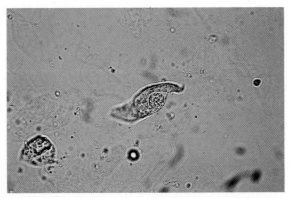

4. Transitional (Caudate) Epithelial Cell, (400X)

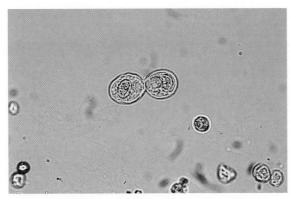

5. Renal Tubular Epithelial Cells and White Blood Cells, (400X)

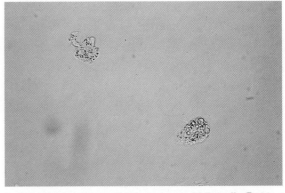

6. Oval Fat Bodies, ×128 (courtesy of Michelle Best, Washington Hospital Center, Washington, D.C.)

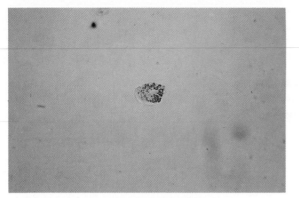

7. Oval Fat Body with Fat Stain, ×128

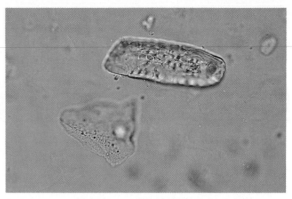

8. Artifact and Squamous Epithelial Cells, (400X)

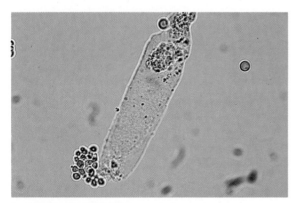

9. Hyaline Cast, (400X)

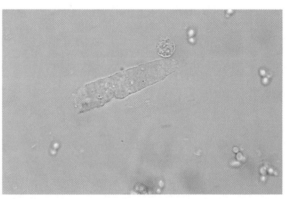

10. Convoluted Hyaline Cast, (400X)

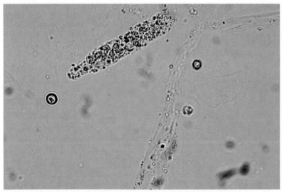

11. Red Blood Cell Cast and Mucus, (400X)

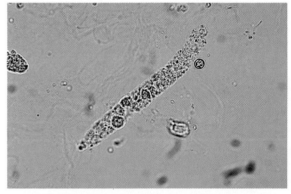

12. White Blood Cell and Granular Cast, (400X)

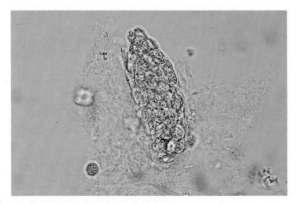

13. Epithelial Cell Cast, (400X)

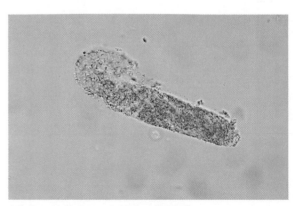

14. Coarsely Granular Cast, (400X)

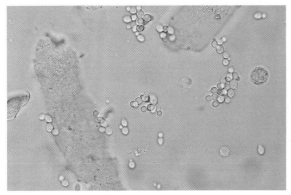

15. Waxy Casts and Yeast, (400X)

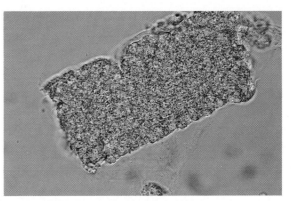

16. Broad Granular Cast, (400X)

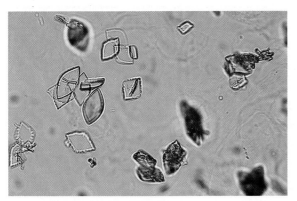

17. Uric Acid Crystals, (400X)

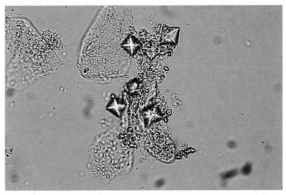

18. Calcium Oxalate Crystals, (400X)

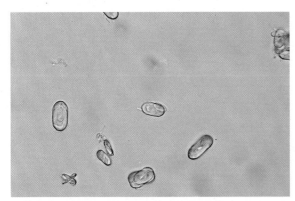

19. Early Calcium Oxalate Crystals, (400X)

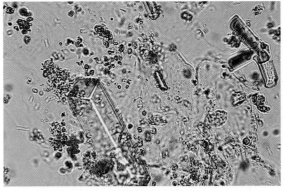

20. Triple Phosphate Crystals, (400X)

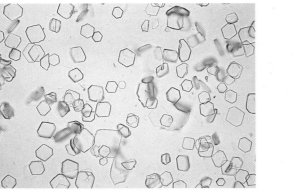

21. Cystine Crystals, ×128 (courtesy of Michelle Best, Washington Hospital Center, Washington, D.C.)

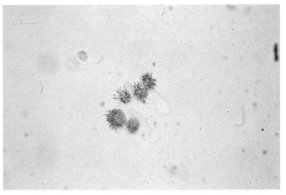

22. Bilirubin Crystals, ×128 (courtesy of Michelle Best, Washington Hospital Center, Washington, D.C.)

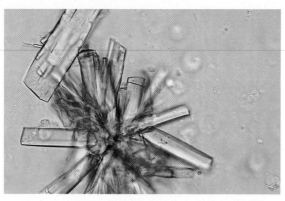

23. Sulfa Crystals, (400X) (courtesy of Michelle Best, Washington Hospital Center, Washington, D.C.)

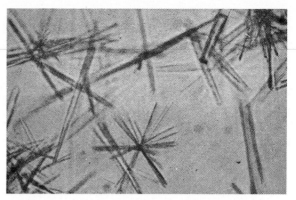

24. Radiographic Dye Crystals, ×128 (courtesy of Michelle Best, Washington Hospital Center, Washington, D.C.)

BODY FLUID CELLS

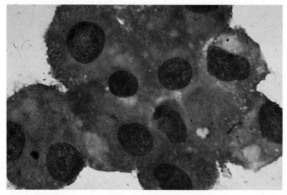

25. Segmented and Pyknotic Neutrophils (CSF), (1000X) (courtesy of The Fairfax Hospital, Fairfax, Virginia)

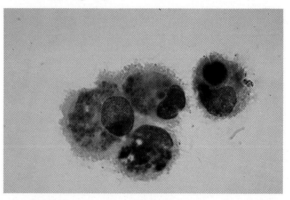

26. Neutrophils, Macrophages, and Mesothelial Cell (CSF), (1000X) (courtesy of The Fairfax Hospital, Fairfax, Virginia)

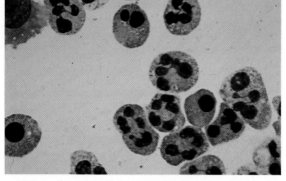

27. Mesothelial Cell Clump (CSF)(1000X)(courtesy of The Fairfax Hospital, Fairfax, Virginia)

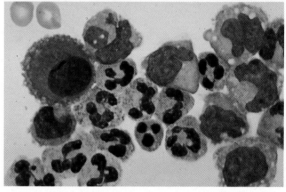

28. Macrophages with Hemosiderin Granules (CSF), (1000X) (courtesy of The Fairfax Hospital, Fairfax, Virginia)

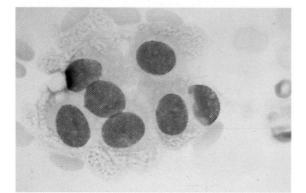

29. Ependymal Cells (CSF), (1000X) (courtesy of The Fairfax Hospital, Fairfax, Virginia)

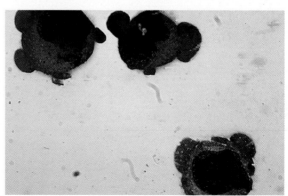

30. Malignant Cells (CSF), (1000X) (courtesy of The Fairfax Hospital, Fairfax, Virginia)

INDEX

A "t" following a page number indicates a table. A page number in *italics* indicates a figure.

Pyronin B, 90
Pyuria, 94

QUALITATIVE fecal fats, 196–197
Quality control
    industrial vs. laboratory, 104t
    methodology of, 105
    of instruments and equipment, 106–107
    of reagents and dipsticks, 105
    personnel and, 108
    routine procedures for, 103–104t
    specimen collection, handling, and
        identification and, 105
Quantitating the microscopic sediment of
    urine, 2
Quantitative fecal fats, 198, 199t

RADIOGRAPHIC dye, 101t, 102
Radiographic dye crystals, Color Plate 24
Radioimmunoassay testing for myoglobin, 71
Ragocytes, 165
    in synovial fluid, 166t
Random specimen, 7
Rapidly progressive glomerulonephritis, 34
Reagents, quality control and, 105
Red blood cell casts, 96–97
Red blood cells, Color Plate 2
    in urine, 43, 93–94
        as cause of turbidity, 45–46
Reducing substances testing, 120t
Refractive index, 48
Refractometer, 48–49
Refractometer scale, 49
Refrigeration, as urine preservative, 4, 5t
Reiter cells, 165
    in synovial fluid, 166t
Renal blood flow, 16–17
Renal blood flow tests, 30–32
Renal calculi, 93
Renal diseases, 32–36
    acute glomerulonephritis, 32, 34
    Addis count and, 89
    cellular casts seen in, 96–97
    chronic glomerulonephritis, 32–33, 34
    focal glomerulonephritis, 33, 34
    hyaline casts in, 96
    laboratory correlations in, 34–35
    membranoproliferative glomerulonephritis,
        33, 34
    membranous glomerulonephritis, 33, 34
    minimal change disease, 33, 35
    nephrotic syndrome, 33, 35, 36
    pyelonephritis, 35, 36
    rapidly progressive glomerulonephritis, 34
    renal failure, 36
    testing for, 2
Renal disorders, vs. overflow disorders, 115,
    116
Renal failure, 36
Renal failure casts, 98
Renal function tests, 22, 23
    clearance tests, 22–25
    Fishberg test, 27
    glomerular filtration, 22–25
    Mosenthal test, 27
    osmolarity measurement and, 27–29

    relationship of nephron areas to, 23
    tubular reabsorption tests, 25–27
    tubular secretion and renal blood flow tests,
        30–32
Renal functions, 15
    glomerular filtration, 17–18, 18
    renal blood flow, 16–17
    tubular reabsorption, 18–20, 19t, 20
Renal graft rejection, 94–95
Renal physiology, 15–22, 15, 16
Renal plasma flow, calculation of, 31
Renal tubular acidosis, 31
Renal tubular cells, 94–95
Renin, 17
Reporting of results, 107, 107t
Reye's syndrome, elevated glutamine test
    and, 146
Rheumatoid arthritis, 169
Rice bodies, seen in synovial fluid, 166t
Ropes viscosity test, 169

SANFILIPPO's syndrome, 126
Schistosoma haematobium, 98
Sediment constituents, 92, 93
    artifacts, 102
    bacteria, 98
    casts, 95–98
    crystals, 98–99, 102
    epithelial cells, 94–95
    mucus, 98
    parasites, 98
    red blood cells, 93–94
    spermatozoa, 98
    staining reactions of, 91–92t
    white blood cells, 94
    yeast, 98
Sediment stains, 90–92, 91–92t
Semen analysis, 158–162
    normal values for, 159t
    testing for abnormal, 162t
Seminal fluid, 158–159
Seminal fluid analysis
    morphology, 160t, 161–162, 161
    motility, 160t, 160–161
    pH, 159, 160t
    viscosity, 159, 160t
    volume, 159, 160t
Seminal fluid fructose level tests, 162, 162t
Septic arthritis, 168, 169
Septic joint disorders, 164t
Serologic examination of cerebrospinal fluid,
    148
Serotonin, 122, 123t
Serous fluids, 169
    formation, 170, 170
    laboratory procedures for examination of,
        171
    peritoneal fluid, 175
    pleural fluid, 172–175
    transudates and exudates, 170–171, 171t,
        172t
Serum osmolarity measurements, 29
Serum protein, 143, 143t
Shake test, 178
Silver-nitroprusside test, 119t
Simulated spinal fluid (SSF), 149–150